THE RAVEN MRI TEACHING FILE

Pediatric MRI

THE RAVEN MRI TEACHING FILE

Pediatric MRI

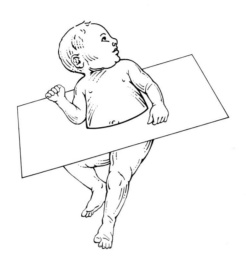

Editor

ROSALIND B. DIETRICH, M.D.

Associate Professor of Radiological Sciences
Director of MRI
University of California, Irvine
Orange, California

RAVEN PRESS ⬡ NEW YORK

Raven Press, 1185 Avenue of the Americas, New York, New York 10036

Made in the United States of America

Library of Congress Cataloging-in-Publication Data

Pediatric MRI/editor, Rosalind Dietrich.
      p.   cm.—(The Raven MRI teaching file)
  Includes bibliographical references.
  Includes in publication.
  ISBN 0-88167-708-6
  1. Children—Diseases—Diagnosis. 2. Magnetic resonance imaging.
 I. Series.
  [DNLM: 1. Diagnosis—in infancy & childhood. 2. Magnetic Resonance Imaging—in infancy & childhood. WS 141 P3679]
  RJ51.M33P43 1991
  618.92'007548—dc20
  DNLM/DLC
  for Library of Congress   91-6875
                                            CIP

9 8 7 6 5 4 3 2 1

To the memory of my father, John Robert Brown.
In loving appreciation of his unfailing support and encouragement.

Preface to the MRI Teaching File

Magnetic Resonance Imaging (MRI) is a complex, rapidly evolving modality which has recently developed applications in all areas of diagnostic radiology. The successful radiologist in the 1990s *must* be proficient at MRI. To develop such proficiency is a formidable task, particularly for radiologists who were not exposed to MRI during their residencies. This 1,000 case MR teaching file is intended to help the practicing radiologist rapidly acquire a storehouse of experience which should aid development of proficiency in MRI. Cases have been carefully selected to show variable manifestations of common pathology as well as the occasional unusual case. The discussions have been kept brief, conforming to the teaching file format. If the reader focuses first on the left hand page while covering the right hand page, retention of information is significantly improved. Although the diagnosis in these workbooks is often suggested by the clinical history and presentation of selected images, the same information of the entire series is available in a convenient single video disk in which the reader is given the option to either choose the selected images reproduced in the printed workbooks or additional images including color and "movie" sequences from the complete imaging file. Additionally, the video disk format allows case presentation either with or without clinical information or orientation to a particular organ system. The video disk is available through Medical Interactive, 3708 Mt. Diablo Boulevard, Suite 120, Lafayette, California 94549.

The series editors would like to thank the section editors for their efforts in organizing the individual 100 case workbooks. This represents contributions from a large number of our friends and colleagues. This also allows us to show cases from a wide variety of manufacturers, MR instruments using a range of magnetic field strengths. We would also like to thank Mary Rogers and her staff at Raven Press for all their help and encouragement during the course of this project.

Robert B. Lufkin, M.D.
William G. Bradley, Jr., M.D., Ph.D.
Michael Brant-Zawadzki, M.D., F.A.C.R.

Although the role of magnetic resonance imaging was quickly established for the evaluation of most organ systems of the adult patient, there has been slower acceptance of its use for the evaluation of the pediatric patient. This is true despite the fact that the combination of direct multiplanar capabilites, superb contrast resolution, and lack of ionizing radiation associated with MRI make it an extremely attractive modality with which to evaluate children.

This book, therefore, has been designed as a MR learning guide and reference manual for radiologists, residents, and clinicians involved in the diagnostic evaluation of children. Thanks to the efforts of the contributing authors, all of whom have extensive experience with MRI and are strong advocates of its use in children, we have attempted to cover in a practical way most of the major indications for the use of magnetic resonance in this patient population.

Rosalind B. Dietrich, M.D.

Acknowledgments

I would like to thank the following people for their enthusiastic contributions, which have added to the quality and diversity of the cases presented in this book: C. Roger Bird, M.D., Richard S. Boyer, M.D., Sharon E. Byrd, M.D., Mervyn D. Cohen, M.B., Ch.B., Sheila G. Moore, M.D., Patricia Perry, M.B., Ch.B., Yutaka Sato, M.D., and Janet L. Strife, M.D.

The Raven MRI Teaching File

Series Editors

Robert B. Lufkin
William G. Bradley, Jr.
Michael Brant-Zawadzki

MRI of the Brain I: Non-Neoplastic Disease
William G. Bradley, Jr. and Michael Brant-Zawadzki, Editors

MRI of the Brain II: Non-Neoplastic Disease
Michael Brant-Zawadzki and William G. Bradley, Jr., Editors

MRI of the Brain III: Neoplastic Disease
Anton N. Hasso, Editor

MRI of the Spine
Robert Quencer, Editor

MRI of the Head and Neck
Robert B. Lufkin and William N. Hanafee, Editors

MRI of the Musculoskeletal System
John V. Crues III, Editor

MRI of the Body
David D. Stark, Editor

MRI of the Cardiovascular System
Rod Pettigrew and Orest Boyko, Editors

Pediatric MRI
Rosalind B. Dietrich, Editor

MRI: Principles and Artifacts
Edward Hendrick, Editor

THE RAVEN MRI TEACHING FILE

Pediatric MRI

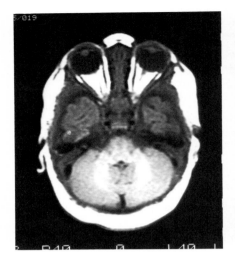

FIG. 1A. SE 600/20.

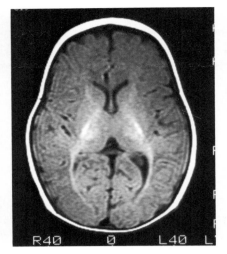

FIG. 1B. SE 600/20.

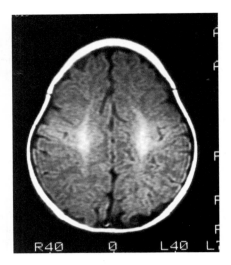

FIG. 1C. SE 600/20.

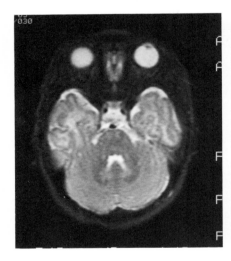

FIG. 1D. SE 3,500/120.

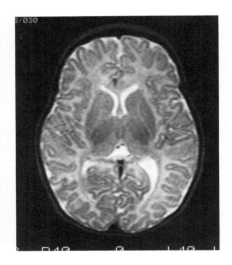

FIG. 1E. SE 3,500/120.

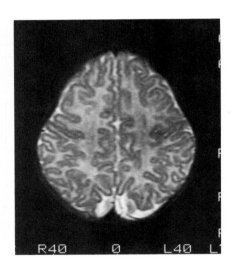

FIG. 1F. SE 3,500/120.

Clinical History

A 2-month-old girl with suspected CNS abnormality on *in utero* ultrasound.

Findings

The cerebral hemispheres demonstrate a mature pattern of sulci and gyri. On T2-weighted images, the signal intensity of the white matter is hyperintense compared to the gray matter. Low signal intensity myelin is seen in the region of the thalamus and in the posterior limb of the internal capsule (Fig. 1E). A small amount of myelin is also present in the optic radiations (Fig. 1E).

On T1-weighted images, the signal intensity of the white matter is hypointense compared to the gray matter. Myelin (which appears white on T1-weighted images) is seen in the same regions described on the T2-weighted images but in addition is also seen in the anterior limb of the internal capsule (Fig. 1B).

Diagnosis

Normal infant brain, infantile pattern.

Discussion

The neonatal brain has a much higher water content than that of the adult and therefore its T1 and T2 values are much longer. During the first 2 years of life, this excess water is gradually lost from both the gray and white matter, but proportionally more is lost from the white matter than from the gray. Therefore, the relative signal intensity of the gray and white matter changes with respect to each other during the first 2 years of life. On T2-weighted images the white matter is normally hyperintense compared to the gray from birth to approximately 8 months of age. On T1-weighted images the white matter is hypointense compared to the gray matter from birth to 3 months of age.

Myelin is a substance consisting of lipid and protein that is laid down around the axons of the CNS by oligodendrocytes. It increases the speed of conduction of nerve impulses along the axons. The deposition of myelin starts during the third trimester of intrauterine life and continues after birth, but the rate of deposition is fastest during the period from birth to 2 years of age. The changes in the appearance of the neonatal brain seen during this time therefore reflect both the loss of water and deposition of myelin.

References

1. Dietrich RB, Bradley WG, Zaragoza EJ, et al. MR evaluation of early myelination patterns in normal and developmentally delayed infants. *AJNR* 1988; 9:69–75.
2. Barkovich AJ, Kjos BO, Jackson DE, Norman D. Normal maturation of the neonatal and infant brain: MR imaging at 1.5T. *Radiology* 1988;166:173–180.

Submitted by: Rosalind B. Dietrich, M.B., Ch.B., Senior Editor.

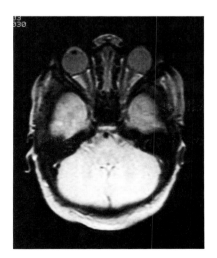

FIG. 1G. SE 3,500/30.

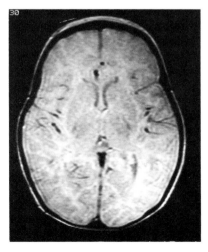

FIG. 1H. SE 3,500/30.

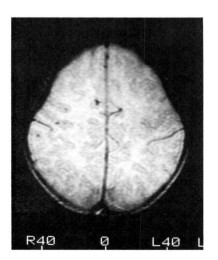

FIG. 1I. SE 3,500/30.

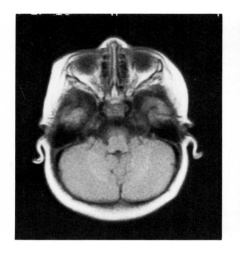

FIG. 2A. SE 800/30.

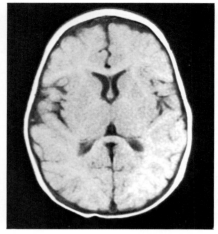

FIG. 2B. SE 800/30.

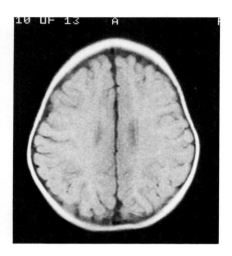

FIG. 2C. SE 800/30.

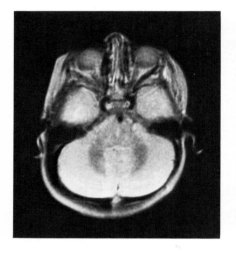

FIG. 2D. SE 2,000/85.

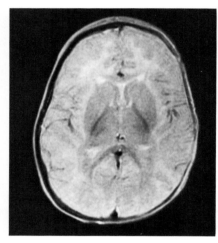

FIG. 2E. SE 2,000/85.

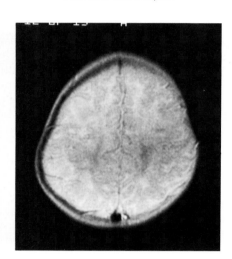

FIG. 2F. SE 2,000/85.

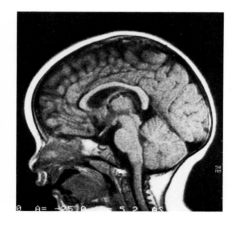

FIG. 2G. SE 500/30.

Clinical History

A 7-month-old child whose sister has CNS malformation.

4

Findings

On T2-weighted images the signal intensity of the white matter is isointense compared to the gray matter in the parietal and occipital areas and hyperintense compared to the gray matter in the frontal lobes. Low signal intensity myelin is present in the thalamus, anterior and posterior limbs of the internal capsule (Fig. 2E), and the centrum semiovale (Fig. 2F). Myelin is also seen in the cerebellar white matter. On T1-weighted images the unmyelinated white and gray matter are isointense; the myelinated white matter has high signal intensity. On sagittal images the corpus callosum has a normal adult appearance (Fig. 2G).

Diagnosis

Normal brain at 7 months.

Discussion

Between the ages of approximately 8 and 12 months, the gray and white matter appear relatively isointense, myelination proceeding from the occipital to the parietal to the frontal to the temporal lobes. Prior to this age, the white matter appears hyperintense compared to the gray. This child, who was 7 months at the time of the scan, demonstrates a transition appearance between the two patterns.

In developmentally normal children, myelin deposition is identified on T2-weighted images in the thalamus at birth, in the posterior limb of the internal capsule at 1 month, in the optic radiations at 3 months, in the anterior limb of the internal capsule at 6 months, and in the white matter of the parietal lobes by 8 months. This child therefore demonstrates a myelin pattern appropriate for age.

References

1. Dietrich RB, Bradley WG, Zaragoza EJ, et al. MR evaluation of early myelination patterns in normal and developmentally delayed infants. *AJNR* 1988; 9:69–75.
2. Barkovich AJ, Kjos BO, Jackson DE, Norman D. Normal maturation of the neonatal and infant brain: MR imaging at 1.5T. *Radiology* 1988;166:173–180.
3. Barkovich AJ, Kjos BO. Normal postnatal development of the corpus callosum as demonstrated by MR imaging. *AJNR* 1988;9:487–491.

Submitted by: Rosalind B. Dietrich, M.B., Ch.B., Senior Editor.

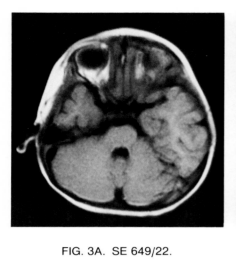

FIG. 3A. SE 649/22.

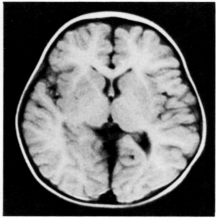

FIG. 3B. SE 649/22.

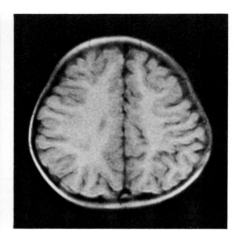

FIG. 3C. SE 649/22.

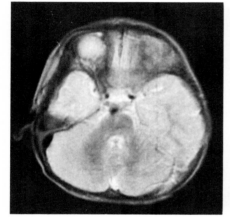

FIG. 3D. SE 3,000/85.

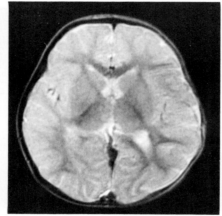

FIG. 3E. SE 3,000/85.

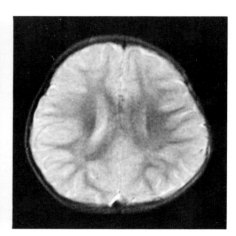

FIG. 3F. SE 3,000/85.

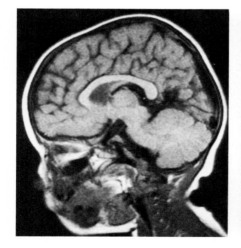

FIG. 3G. SE 374/30.

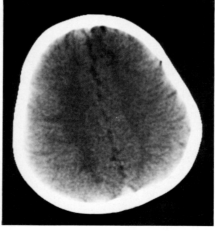

FIG. 3H. CT.

Clinical History

A 12-month-old girl with a border-line-high head circumference.

6

Findings

CT scan without contrast demonstrates that the density of the white matter is lower than that of the gray. No abnormalities are seen. On MR images, the sulci and gyri appear normal. On T2-weighted images the signal intensity of the white matter is hypointense compared to the gray matter. Myelin deposition is seen not only centrally in the regions of the internal capsule and optic radiations but is also extending peripherally throughout the white matter to the subcortical U-fibers (Figs. 3E and F). There are discrete areas of higher signal intensity within the white matter dorsal and superior to the ventricular trigones (Fig. 3F). On T1-weighted spin-echo and inversion recovery images the myelinated white matter has higher signal intensity than the adjacent gray matter. On sagittal T1-weighted images the corpus callosum is normally formed and has higher signal intensity than the adjacent brain parenchyma due to myelin deposition within it (Fig. 3G).

Diagnosis

Normal brain at 12 months.

Discussion

By 12 months of age the relative signal intensities of the gray and white matter of the pediatric brain are the same as those of the adult. At this time, the deposition of myelin is present in the white matter both centrally and peripherally. The process of myelination within the brain continues until at least the early twenties, and there is now evidence to suggest that it continues to occur throughout life. The rate of myelin deposition, however, is much slower after 2 years of age.

References

1. Dietrich RB, Bradley WG, Zaragoza EJ, et al. MR evaluation of early myelination patterns in normal and developmentally delayed infants. *AJNR* 1988; 9:69–75.
2. Barkovich AJ, Kjos BO, Jackson DE, Norman D. Normal maturation of the neonatal and infant brain: MR imaging at 1.5T. *Radiology* 1988;166:173–180.
3. Barkovich AJ, Kjos BO. Normal postnatal development of the corpus callosum as demonstrated by MR imaging. *AJNR* 1988;9:487–491.

Submitted by: Rosalind B. Dietrich, M.B., Ch.B., Senior Editor.

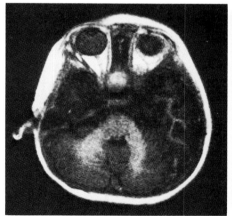 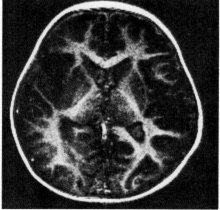 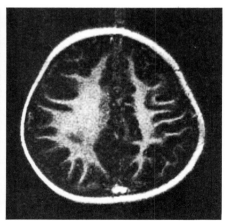

FIG. 3I. IR 1,500/300/30.   FIG. 3J. IR 1,500/300/30.   FIG. 3K. IR 1,500/300/30.

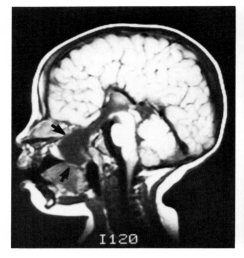

FIG. 4A. SE 500/20.

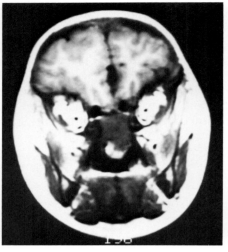

FIG. 4B. SE 500/20.

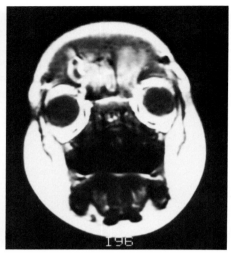

FIG. 4C. SE 500/20.

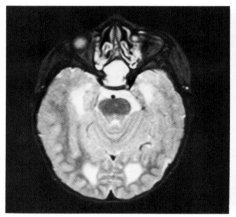

FIG. 4D. SE 2,500/80.

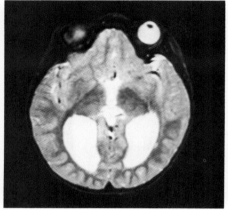

FIG. 4E. SE 2,500/80.

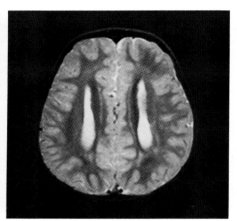

FIG. 4F. SE 2,500/80.

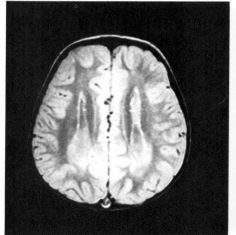

FIG. 4G. SE 2,500/30.

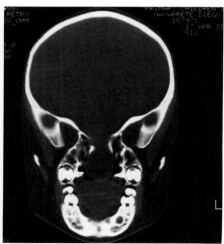

FIG. 4H. CT.

Clinical History

A 2-year-old male from South America with hypertelorism was noted to have a mass in the oropharynx posterior to a cleft palate.

Findings

The midline sagittal T1- and axial T2-weighted scans (Figs. 4A and D) show a defect in the sphenoid bone with herniation of a CSF-filled structure through the sphenoid bone defect into the naso- and oropharynx (*arrows*). This sac is in continuity with the floor of the third ventricle via the infundibular recess. Also noted is agenesis of the corpus callosum and enlargement of the atrial and occipital portions of the lateral ventricles (colpocephaly) (Figs. 4A, D, and E). Direct coronal CT scans with bone window images confirm the large bone defect in the sphenoid bone at the level of the anterior clinoids (Fig. 4H). Interestingly, the majority of the cribiform plate is intact, although misshapen, and the crista galli is not well formed.

Diagnosis

Nasosphenoid encephalocele with herniation of the third ventricle into the naso-oropharynx.

Discussion

Encephaloceles are congenital malformations in which the brain, ventricles, and/or overlying meninges protrude outside the cranial cavity via a defect in bone or soft tissue. They are most commonly found in the occipital (71%), parietal (10%), frontal (9%), nasal (9%), and sphenoid (2%) regions. They may also be off the midline at the pterion or asterion. If no brain protrudes through the defect, the lesion is more properly termed a "cephalocele" or a "cephalic meningocele." In this case, even though only a CSF-filled structure protrudes through the sphenoid defect, because this is a portion of the third ventricle, the correct diagnosis is encephalocele.

Associated features may include agenesis of the corpus callosum, abnormalities of gyration and sulcation, and schizencephaly. Low occipital and/or upper cervical encephaloceles associated with hindbrain herniation are termed "Chiari III malformation."

Reference

1. Naidich TP, Zimmerman RA. Common congenital malformations of the brain. In: Brant-Zawadzki M, Norman D, eds. *Magnetic resonance imaging of the central nervous system.* New York: Raven Press, 1987;131–150.

Submitted by: Richard S. Boyer, M.D., Primary Children's Medical Center, Salt Lake City, Utah; Rosalind B. Dietrich, M.B., Ch.B., Senior Editor.

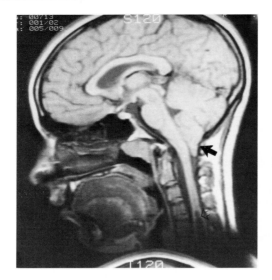

FIG. 5A. SE 600/20.

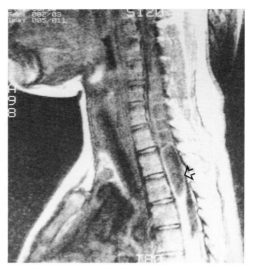

FIG. 5B. SE 800/20.

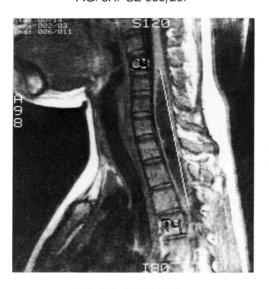

FIG. 5C. SE 800/20.

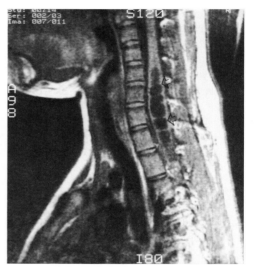

FIG. 5D. SE 800/20.

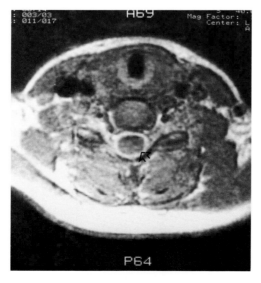

FIG. 5E. SE 1,500/20.

Clinical History

A 16-year-old female, 2 years status post-neck injury with increasing weakness and sensory loss in arms.

10

Findings

Sagittal scans of the brain show tonsilar herniation (Fig. 5A, *arrow*) with normal posterior fossa structures, brain stem, and supratentorial structures. The sagittal brain images show the upper portion of the syrinx beginning at the lower margin of C4. There is no hydrocephalus present. Sagittal and axial images of the spine identify a fluid-filled cyst within the spinal cord extending from the lower margin of C4 to the upper margin of T4. Multiple transverse internal septations are seen within the cystic cavity (Figs. 5B–E, *open arrows*).

Diagnosis

Chiari I.

Discussion

Chiari described four types of unrelated cerebellar malformations. Chiari I malformation, which is unrelated to Chiari II malformation, is characterized by herniation of the inferior cerebellar tonsils through the foramen magnum into the upper cervical spinal canal. It is thought to be a dysplasia of the cervical and occipital bones and sometimes called "tonsillar ectopia." Cranial and skeletal anomalies are uncommon, and it is not associated with a myelomeningocele, although syringohydromyelia or hydromyelia are associated in 60%–70% of cases. Associated conditions include basilar invagination, Klippel-Feil, and assimilation of C1 to the occiput. It is usually asymptomatic, although some cases present with headache, raised intracranial pressure, and/or hydrocephalus. Three syndromes that are symptomatic in older children and adults include (a) foramen magnum compression with ataxia, corticospinal and sensory deficits, cerebellar signs, and lower cranial nerve deficits; (b) central cord syndrome with combined, dissociated sensory loss; and (c) cerebellar syndrome with truncal ataxia, nystagmus, and limb ataxia.

MR findings include malformed craniovertebral junction with basilar impression, assimilation of C1 to the occiput, partial fusions C2–3, Klippel-Feil deformity, cervical dysraphism, widening of cervical spinal canal from hydromyelia, and caudal elongation of tonsils through the foramen magnum. The tonsils may be asymmetric in size and position. Other features include small cisterna magna, syringohydromyelia of the cervical cord, and hydrocephalus.

Reference

1. Byrd SE, Osborn RE, Radkowski MA, et al. Disorders of midline structures: holoprosencephaly, absence of corpus callosum and Chiari malformations. *Semin US CT MR* 1988;9:201–215.

Submitted by: Arthur Watanabe, M.D., and Richard S. Boyer, M.D., Primary Children's Medical Center, Salt Lake City, Utah; Rosalind B. Dietrich, M.B., Ch.B., Senior Editor.

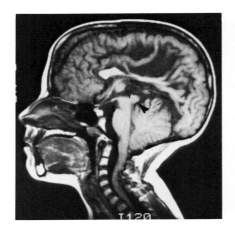

FIG. 6A. SE 600/20.

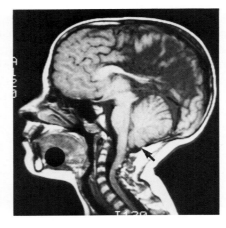

FIG. 6B. SE 600/20.

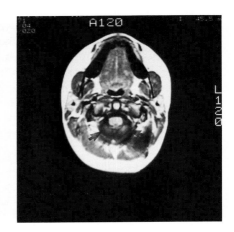

FIG. 6C. SE 800/20.

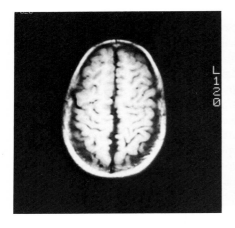

FIG. 6D. SE 800/20.

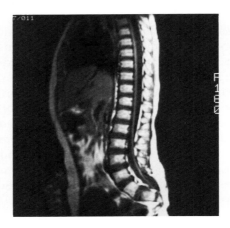

FIG. 6E. SE 600/20.

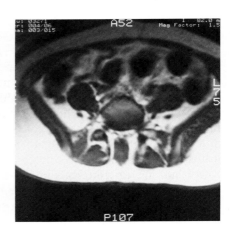

FIG. 6F. SE 800/30.

Clinical History

A 9-year-old female born with lumbosacral meningomyelocele. An intraventricular shunt catheter was placed for hydrocephalus.

Findings

Sagittal and axial T1-weighted imaging of the brain demonstrates a small posterior fossa with downward displacement of the brain stem and cerebellum through the foramen magnum (although not as severely herniated as in many cases) (Figs. 6A–C, *arrow*). There are upward protrusion of the vermis through the tentorial incisura, beaking of the tectum (Figs. 6A and B, *arrowhead*), prominent massa intermedia (Fig. 6A, *open arrow*), dysplastic corpus callosum, incomplete falx with interdigitation of the gyri, shunted hydrocephalus, and small, closely spaced gyri (stenogyria) (Fig. 6D). Sagittal and axial T1-weighted images of the spine demonstrate distal spinal dysraphism with extension of the spinal cord into the dysraphic defect, without an identifiable conus (Figs. 6E and F). The distal cord may be tethered at the site of meningomyelocele repair. No syrinx, lipoma, or dermoid is seen.

Diagnosis

Chiari II malformation with shunted hydrocephalus.

Discussion

Chiari described four types of unrelated cerebellar malformations. Chiari II is a complex disorder of closure malformation that affects the calvarium, dura, and hindbrain. It is almost always associated with myelomeningocele. Incidence is estimated at 3/1,000 births with a female predominance 2:1. Patients present with a myelomeningocele and have sensory and motor deficits of the lower extremities, hydrocephalus, and increased intracranial pressure.

MR findings are complex and numerous. Multiple abnormalities characterize this malformation. The disorder is best thought of as "hindbrain dysgenesis." There is herniation of the hindbrain (brain stem and cerebellum) through the enlarged foramen magnum into the upper cervical canal. Fixation of the upper cervical cord produces a medullary kink of the brain stem below the level of the foramen magnum. The fourth ventricle is compressed and displaced caudally. The vermis may herniate upwardly through the tentorial incisura, producing beaking of the inferior portion of the quadrigeminal plate. Other features of the brain malformation include dysplastic changes of the corpus callosum, incomplete falx, and a disordering of the gyral pattern, incorrectly termed "polymicrogyria." This is better described as "stenogyria," meaning closely spaced, small gyri. Pathologically these have a full six-layer cortex and therefore do not fit in the pachygyria-polymicrogyria spectrum. Hydrocephalus is almost always a feature of Chiari II malformation. The obstruction is at the level of the aqueduct but may relate to the tight incisura. Many of the features of Chiari II malformation are better seen after shunting of the hydrocephalus.

Reference

1. Byrd SE, Osborn RE, Radkowski MA, et al. Disorders of midline structures: holoprosencephaly, absence of corpus callosum and Chiari malformations. *Semin US CT MR* 1988;9:201–215.

Submitted by: Arthur Watanabe, M.D., and Richard S. Boyer, M.D., Primary Children's Medical Center, Salt Lake City, Utah; Rosalind B. Dietrich, M.B., Ch.B., Senior Editor.

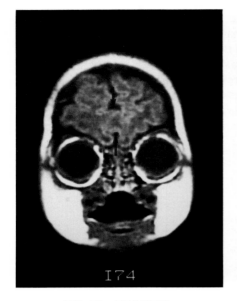

FIG. 7A. SE 600/20.

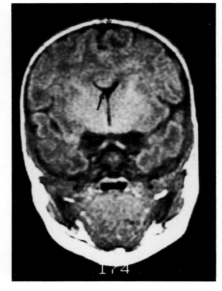

FIG. 7B. SE 600/20.

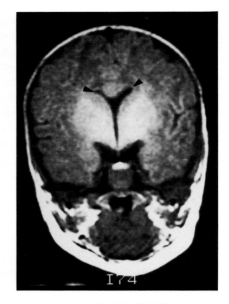

FIG. 7C. SE 600/20.

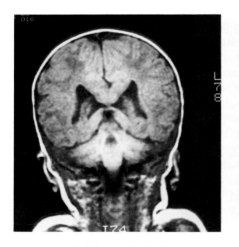

FIG. 7D. SE 600/20.

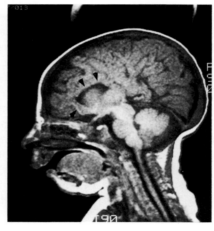

FIG. 7E. SE 600/20.

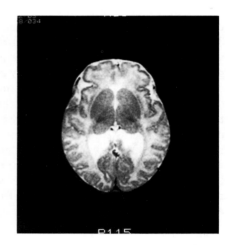

FIG. 7F. SE 4,000/100.

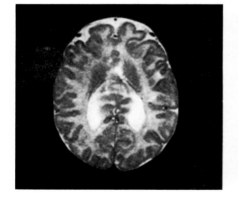

FIG. 7G. SE 4,000/100.

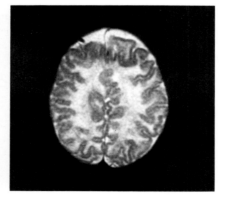

FIG. 7H. SE 4,000/100.

Clinical History

A 1-month-old male, product of an uncomplicated pregnancy and cesarean delivery, has a family history of agenesis of the corpus callosum.

Findings

The coronal T1-weighted images demonstrate fusion of the frontal lobes anteriorly with partial absence of the anterior portions of the falx cerebri and interhemispheric fissure (Figs. 7A and B, *arrows*). The frontal horns are somewhat blunted with squared lateral margins (Fig. 7C, *arrowheads*). The septum pellucidum is absent. The corpus callosum is present but is difficult to differentiate from the adjacent nonmyelinated white matter. This is a normal finding in a child of 1 month (Fig. 7E, *small arrowheads*). There is slight prominence to the occipital and temporal horns of the lateral ventricles. There is normal development of the parietal, occipital, and temporal lobes. The third ventricle is well visualized and appears unremarkable with a cleaved thalamus. Age-appropriate reversal of the gray-white matter signal intensity in the T2-weighted images is noted consistent with an immature myelin pattern (Figs. 7F–H). The remainder of the examination is unremarkable. Note the excellent gray/white differentiation on the SE(4,000/100) images.

Diagnosis

Lobar holoprosencephaly.

Discussion

Holoprosencephaly is a spectrum of congenital midline malformations caused by partial to complete failure of diverticulation of the prosencephalon (forebrain). This malformation is thought to occur between 4 and 8 weeks of gestation. Holoprosencephaly is typically categorized as alobar, semilobar, or lobar depending on the degree of forebrain cleavage. Some consider septo-optic dysplasia (de Morsier's syndrome) as the mildest form of the holoprosencephaly syndrome. Lobar holoprosencephaly is the least severe form. The brain undergoes nearly complete cleavage, forming parietal, occipital, and temporal lobes with fusion limited to the frontal lobes anteriorly. Holoprosencephaly is associated with midline facial dysmorphism ranging from hypotelorism and cleft palate to cyclops.

The clinical presentation of holoprosencephaly is variable with dysmorphic facies, microcephaly, seizures, developmental delay, and mental retardation, the most common presenting features. Occasionally patients will present with macrocephaly and, therefore, must be differentiated from patients with hydrocephalus.

The MR features of lobar holoprosencephaly include partial fusion of the frontal lobes with absence of the anterior portion of the falx cerebri and interhemispheric fissure. The frontal horns are blunted and squared off laterally. The septum pellucidum is absent. The corpus callosum is usually present, although it may be diminutive anteriorly. The temporal, parietal, and occipital lobes form normally. In distinction to the alobar and semilobar forms of holoprosencephaly, the third ventricle is normal without thalamic fusion.

References

1. Byrd SE, Osborn RE, Radkowski MA, et al. Disorders of midline structures: holoprosencephaly, absence of corpus callosum, and Chiari malformations. *Semin US CT MR* 1988;9:201–215.
2. Nyberg DA, Mack LA, Bronstein A, et al. Holoprosencephaly: prenatal sonographic diagnosis. *AJNR* 1987;8:871–878.
3. Fitz CR. Holoprosencephaly and related entities. *Neuroradiology* 1983;25:226–238.

Submitted by: Wayne Davis, M.D., and Richard S. Boyer, M.D., Primary Children's Medical Center, Salt Lake City, Utah; Rosalind B. Dietrich, M.B., Ch.B., Senior Editor.

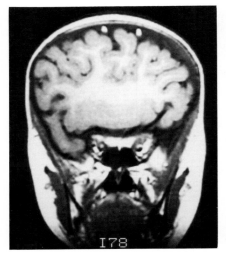

FIG. 8A. SE 800/20.

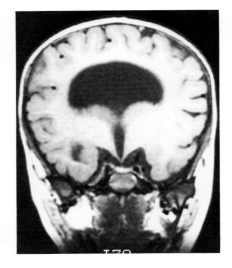

FIG. 8B. SE 800/20.

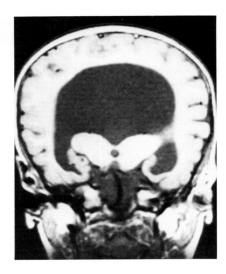

FIG. 8C. SE 800/20.

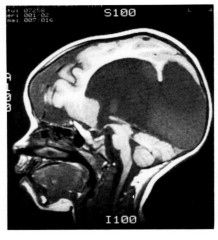

FIG. 8D. SE 600/20.

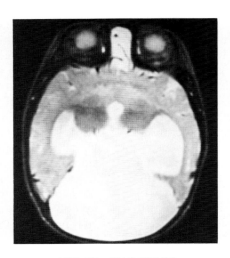

FIG. 8E. SE 2,500/80.

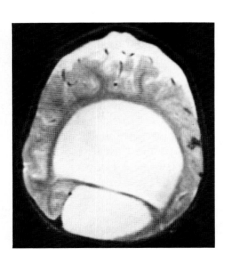

FIG. 8F. SE 2,500/80.

Clinical History

A 23-month-old female with hypotelorism but no other facial midline malformation.

Findings

Multiplanar MR images demonstrate the absence of the falx and interhemispheric fissure (Figs. 8A–C). There is a large anterior monoventricle present and no corpus callosum (Fig. 8D). Posteriorly, there is a dorsal midline cyst. However, the occipital and temporal portions of the ventricles are identifiable (Fig. 8E), and there is partial cleaving of the thalami and a partially formed third ventricle (Figs. 8B and E). The brain stem and cerebellum are small (Fig. 8D). The sagittal sinus and straight sinus are rudimentary, if present. A single midline anterior cerebral artery (ACA) probably represents an azygos variation of the ACA (Fig. 8F). Increased extraaxial fluid is seen anterior to the fused frontal lobes (Fig. 8D).

Diagnosis

Semilobar holoprosencephaly.

Discussion

Holoprosencephaly is a spectrum of cerebral malformations characterized by microcephaly, hypotelorism, and failure to form separate left and right cerebral hemispheres or thalami. Alobar holoprosencephaly is the extreme form of holoprosencephaly resulting in a single horseshoe-shaped supratentorial ventricle with thin cortical tissue. The thalami are fused. The third ventricle, which is unidentifiable, is incorporated into the single ventricle. The septum pellucidum and the interhemispheric fissure are absent. Associated abnormalities include facial anomalies (cleft lip and palate), microphthalmia, anophthalmia, micrognathia, or trigonocephaly. Trisomy 13–15, 18, 18p-, and 13q-syndromes are known associations. Infants with alobar holoprosencephaly do not usually survive.

In semilobar holoprosencephaly, there is an attempt at formation of the lobes of the brain with some cleaving of the thalamus and formation of the third ventricle. In lobar holoprosencephaly, the thalamus cleaves and the hemispheres are better formed. The falx is partially present with some formation of interhemispheric fissure and the corpus callosum is usually detectable. These children have the best prognosis in the spectrum.

Reference

1. Byrd SE, Osborn RE, Radkowski MA, et al. Disorders of midline structures: holoprosencephaly, absence of corpus callosum and Chiari malformations. *Semin US CT MR* 1988;9:201–215.

Submitted by: Arthur Watanabe, M.D., and Richard S. Boyer, M.D., Primary Children's Medical Center, Salt Lake City, Utah; Rosalind B. Dietrich, M.B., Ch.B., Senior Editor.

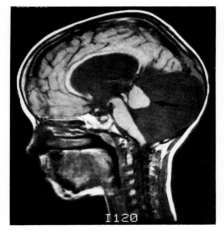

FIG. 9A. SE 600/20.

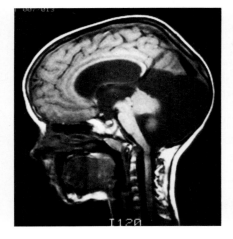

FIG. 9B. SE 600/20.

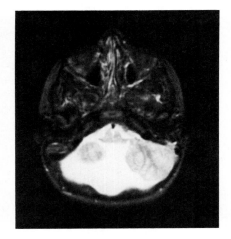

FIG. 9C. SE 2,500/80.

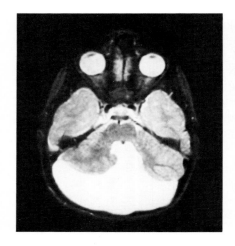

FIG. 9D. SE 2,500/80.

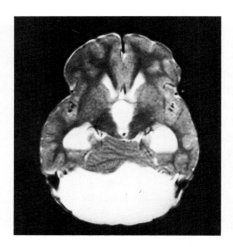

FIG. 9E. SE 2,500/80.

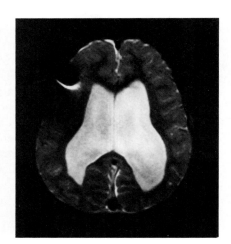

FIG. 9F. SE 2,500/80.

Clinical History

A 5-year-old female with a history of unknown head injury with vomiting and right facial palsy.

Findings

The sagittal scans show that there is only a small amount of superior vermis present (Fig. 9A, *arrow*). The majority of the vermis is absent, allowing communication between the fourth ventricle and a large posterior fossa cyst that elevates the torcular (Fig. 9B). The cerebral aqueduct is open (Fig. 9A, *arrowhead*). There is moderate dilatation of the third and lateral ventricles with a right lateral ventricular shunt catheter in place (Figs. 9E and F). The cerebellar hemispheres are partially compressed by the posterior fossa cysts or bilaterally hypoplastic (Figs. 9C and D). The corpus callosum is thinned by enlargement of the third ventricle (Fig. 9A).

Diagnosis

Dandy-Walker malformation.

Discussion

Dandy-Walker malformation is a dysgenesis of the cerebellar roof resulting in a cystic malformation of the posterior fossa and a large CSF space posterior to the cerebellum. It is characterized by the absence of the vermis and the foramen of Magendie and marked dilatation of the fourth ventricle to form a cyst posterior to the cerebellum. Dysgenesis of the corpus callosum is the most frequently noted coexisting anomaly. Clinically, the patients may present with seizures, developmental delay, and enlarging head size. Recently, some authors proposed that the Dandy-Walker malformation, Dandy-Walker variant, and megacisterna magna may represent a continuum of developmental anomalies of the posterior fossa.

MRI findings include macrocephaly with hydrocephalus, expansion of posterior fossa with scaphocephaly and scalloping of the petrous pyramids, high insertion of the tentorium above the lambda ("torcular-lambda inversion") with wide, more vertically oriented incisura, absent inferior vermis, variably persistent superior vermis displaced superiorly and anteriorly into the incisura by the dilated fourth ventricle and cyst, hypoplastic cerebellar hemispheres, and ballooning of the fourth ventricle into a retrocerebellar cyst that displaces the cerebellar hemispheres against the petrous pyramids.

References

1. Fitz CR. Disorders of ventricles and CSF spaces. *Semin US CT MR* 1988;9:216–230.
2. Barkovich AJ, Kjos BO, Norman D, et al. Revised classification of posterior fossa cysts and cystlike malformations based on the results of multiplanar MR imaging. *AJNR* 1989;10:977–988.

Submitted by: Arthur Watanabe, M.D., and Richard S. Boyer, M.D., Primary Children's Medical Center, Salt Lake City, Utah; Rosalind B. Dietrich, M.B., Ch.B., Senior Editor.

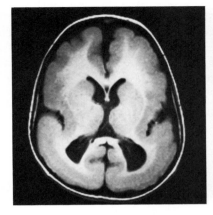

FIG. 10A. SE 800/20.

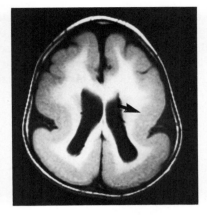

FIG. 10B. SE 800/20.

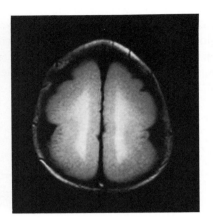

FIG. 10C. SE 800/20.

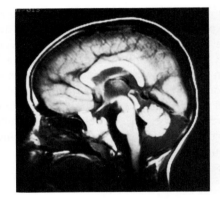

FIG. 10D. SE 600/20.

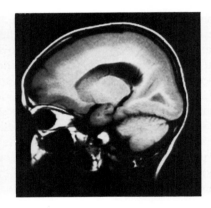

FIG. 10E. SE 600/20.

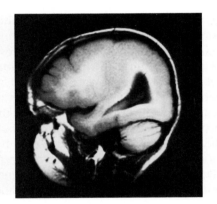

FIG. 10F. SE 600/20.

Clinical History

A 6-year-old male with severe developmental delay and seizures since birth.

Findings

The T1-weighted axial, coronal, and sagittal images demonstrate a smooth cerebral cortex in the parietal and occipital areas with early sulcation and broad flat gyri noted in the frontal and anterior temporal regions. The gray matter of the cortex is thickened (Fig. 10B, *arrow*) with a smooth gray-white interface. There is moderate ventricular enlargement. The midline structures including the corpus callosum and septum pellucidum appear unremarkable. T2-weighted axial scans show similar findings.

Diagnosis

Lissencephaly (agyria).

Discussion

Lissencephaly is a rare congenital brain malformation that is part of the spectrum of diseases of migration and sulcation. Lissencephaly, in the strict sense, means agyria (smooth brain); however, in practical terms, it is used to represent a spectrum of diseases ranging from agyria to agyria with mixed areas of pachygyria (broad, flat gyri). Pathologically, instead of finding a normal six-layered cortex, a four-layered cortex is seen with areas of pachygyria and polymicrogyria. Lissencephaly has multiple causes including genetic (Norman-Roberts and Neu-Larova), chromosomal (Miller-Dieker), infectious, and idiopathic.

Patients typically present with severe developmental delay and seizures. A number of the above-mentioned syndromes have characteristic facial features. Severe forms of lissencephaly are associated with early neonatal death. The isolated idiopathic form of lissencephaly is typically associated with the longest life span, as long as 6–7 years.

The MR features of lissencephaly include a brain surface that is agyric (smooth), with or without areas of pachygyria. The brain assumes an hourglass configuration due to the lack of opercularization of the brain. The sylvian fissure has a primitive vertical orientation and the temporal lobes are small. The cerebral cortex is markedly thickened with an abnormal gray/white matter ratio and lack of normal gray-white matter interdigitation. Other features include enlarged ventricles and variable hypoplasia of the corpus callosum.

References

1. Byrd SE, Bohan TP, Osborn RE, et al. The CT and MR evaluation of lissencephaly. *AJNR* 1988;9:923–927.
2. Lee BCP. MR of lissencephaly. *AJNR* 1988;9:804.
3. Barkovich AJ, Chuang SH, Norman D. MR of neuronal migration anomalies. *AJNR* 1987;8:1009–1017.

Submitted by: Wayne Davis, M.D., and Richard S. Boyer, M.D., Primary Children's Medical Center, Salt Lake City, Utah; Rosalind B. Dietrich, M.B., Ch.B., Senior Editor.

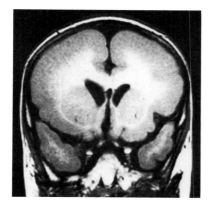

FIG. 10G. SE 800/20.

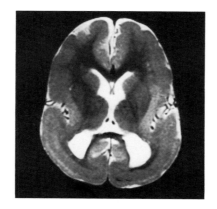

FIG. 10H. SE 2,500/80.

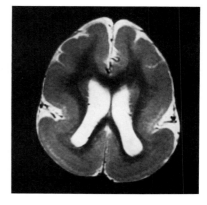

FIG. 10I. SE 2,500/80.

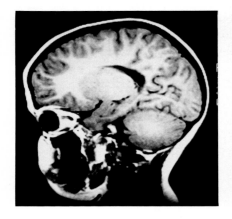

FIG. 11A. SE 500/20.

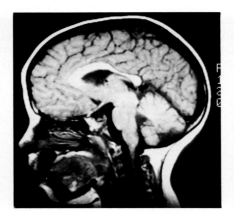

FIG. 11B. SE 500/20.

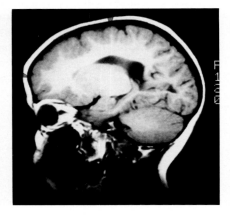

FIG. 11C. SE 500/20.

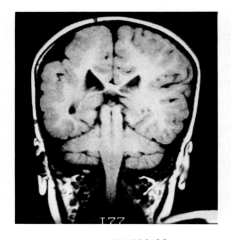

FIG. 11D. SE 700/20.

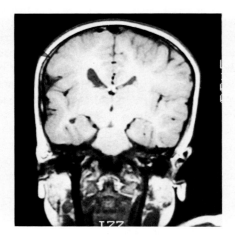

FIG. 11E. SE 700/20.

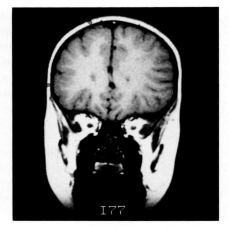

FIG. 11F. SE 700/20.

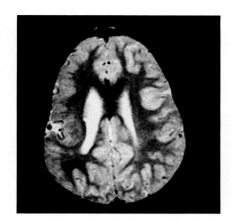

FIG. 11G. SE 2,500/80.

Clinical History

A 6-year-old male with developmental delay, abnormal EEG patterns, and new onset generalized tonic-clonic seizures.

Findings

Pachygyria is present in the right anterior and midparietal region with an abnormal column of gray matter seen in this region extending almost to the ventricular surface (Figs. 11C–F, *arrows*). Abnormal venous drainage is present at the periphery of the area of pachygyria. Mild dilatation of the right lateral ventricle, particularly in the atrium and occipital horn, is seen (Figs. 11D and E).

Diagnosis

Pachygyria.

Discussion

MRI clearly distinguishes between the brain's gray and white matter. Pachygyria falls within the spectrum of neuronal migration anomalies, which also include agyria, polymicrogyria, unilateral megalencephaly, schizencephaly, and gray matter heterotopias. This broad group of anomalies is characterized by ectopic location of neurons in the cerebral cortex. Syndromes with lissencephaly (smooth brain) include agyria (absence of cortical gyri) and pachygyria. Pachygyria, which may be focal or diffuse, is typified by broad gyri, four cortical layers, and few sulci. It has been associated with the presence of laminar heterotopic gray matter. Patients usually present with seizures, developmental delay, or mental retardation. MR demonstrates thickened gray matter in the pachygyria/agyria complex with reversal of the normal gray-white ratio. Cortical convolutions and gray-white interfaces are smoother than normal and the subcortical white matter is thinned. Other associated anomalies may include small brain stem, heterotopias, polymicrogyria, midline malformations, schizencephaly, and inflammatory processes. Pachygyric cortex may have draining vascular channels that mimic vascular malformations.

References

1. Smith AS, Ross JS, Blaser SI, et al. Magnetic resonance imaging of disturbances in neuronal migration: illustration of an embryologic process. *Radiographics* 1989;9:509.
2. Barkovich AJ. Abnormal vascular drainage in anomalies of neuronal migration. *AJNR* 1988;9:939–942.
3. Pollei SR, Boyer RS, Crawford S, et al. Disorders of migration and sulcation. *Semin US CT MR* 1988;9:231–246.

Submitted by: Arthur Watanabe, M.D., and Richard S. Boyer, M.D., Primary Children's Medical Center, Salt Lake City, Utah; Rosalind B. Dietrich, M.B., Ch.B., Senior Editor.

23

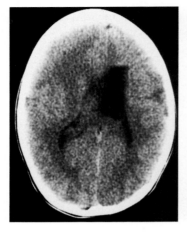

FIG. 12A. CT.

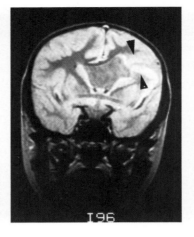

FIG. 12B. SE 2,500/30.

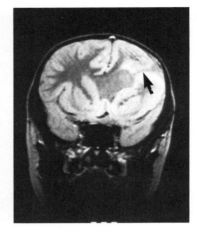

FIG. 12C. SE 2,500/30.

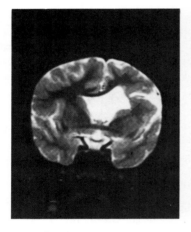

FIG. 12D. SE 2,500/80.

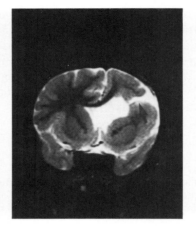

FIG. 12E. SE 2,500/80.

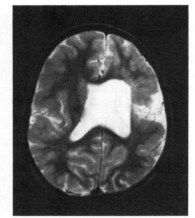

FIG. 12F. SE 2,500/80.

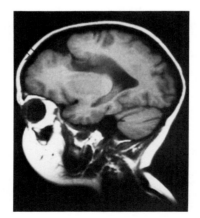

FIG. 12G. SE 500/20.

Clinical History

A 7-year-old male with seizures and developmental delay.

24

Findings

There is asymmetry of the lateral ventricles with dilatation of the left lateral ventricle identified (Figs. 12D, E, and F). There is an area of CSF signal intensity extending from the left frontal subarachnoid space into the lateral margin of the left lateral ventricle (Figs. 12C and E, *arrows*). This CSF-filled cleft is bordered by gray matter signal intensity consistent with open lip schizencephaly (Fig. 12B, *arrowheads*). There is enlargement of the gyri in the left frontal region and the sulci are fewer than expected consistent with pachygyria (Figs. 12E and F). No septum pellucidum is identified. The remainder of the midline structures are unremarkable.

Diagnosis

Open lip schizencephaly.

Discussion

Schizencephaly is a term originally introduced by Yakolev to describe "bilateral, nearly symmetric full-thickness clefts within the cerebral hemispheres." Since the time of Yakolev's description, it has become apparent that schizencephaly is a spectrum of brain malformations ranging from small unilateral clefts to large bilateral clefts. It is classified into two forms: "open" and "closed" lip schizencephaly. In open lip schizencephaly, the cleft extends from the subarachnoid space to the ventricle and is filled with CSF. The closed lip variety presents as a column of gray matter from the subarachnoid space to the ventricle without communication of CSF. In both types of schizencephaly, the cleft is lined by gray matter, identified pathologically as a continual connection of the pia mater to the ependymal lining, the so-called pia-ependymal seam. Associated abnormalities seen in schizencephaly include other areas of gray matter heterotopia, pachygyria, and absence of the septum pellucidum.

The cause of schizencephaly is unknown. It is thought to relate to destruction of a portion of the germinal matrix secondary to ischemia in the seventh week of gestation. The patients present with a broad range of clinical features from normal intelligence to severe developmental delay and disability. Most patients have a seizure disorder that is sometimes intractable. The severity of disease roughly correlates with the extent of schizencephaly, i.e., patients with unilateral clefts are typically less affected than patients with large bilateral clefts.

MRI is exquisitely sensitive to schizencephaly. It is far better than CT secondary to its multiplanar capability and gray-white discrimination. In schizencephaly, MR demonstrates a column of gray matter signal intensity extending from the cortex to the lateral ventricle. In open lip schizencephaly, CSF signal intensity is seen extending from the subarachnoid space to the ventricle. In closed lip schizencephaly, gray matter columns are seen extending from the cortex to the ventricle; however, a complete column of CSF signal intensity is not identified. Many times a small diverticulum is seen in the lateral ventricle at the level of the cleft. One must also look for associated abnormalities, which include pachygyria, gray matter heterotopias, and absent septum pellucidum. In addition to these findings, hypoplasia of the optic nerves has been reported.

The major differential diagnosis is porencephaly, which is a CSF-filled space connected to the ventricle, thought to be related to a destructive process. Porencephaly can be differentiated from schizencephaly by the lack of gray matter lining the porencephalic cyst.

References

1. Barkovich AJ, Norman D. MR imaging of schizencephaly. *AJNR* 1987;9:297–302.
2. Bird CR, Gilles FH. Type I schizencephaly: CT and neuropathologic findings. *AJNR* 1987;8:451–454.

Submitted by: Wayne Davis, M.D., and Richard S. Boyer, M.D., Primary Children's Medical Center, Salt Lake City, Utah; Rosalind B. Dietrich, M.B., Ch.B., Senior Editor.

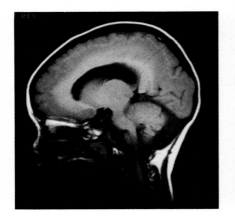

FIG. 13A. SE 500/20.

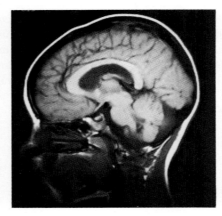

FIG. 13B. SE 500/20.

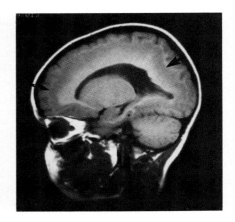

FIG. 13C. SE 500/20.

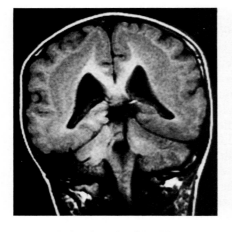

FIG. 13D. SE 600/20.

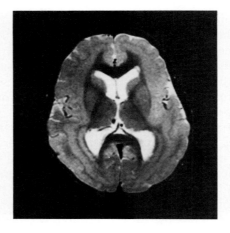

FIG. 13E. SE 2,500/80.

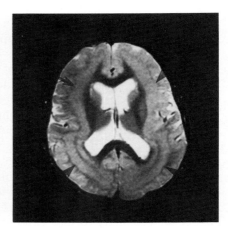

FIG. 13F. SE 2,500/80.

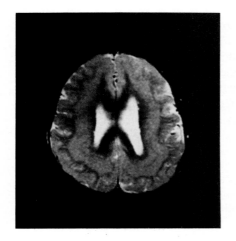

FIG. 13G. SE 2,500/80.

Clinical History

A 4-year-old white female with seizures and developmental delay.

26

Findings

The sagittal and coronal T1-weighted images demonstrate intermediate signal intensity, the same as that of the cortical gray matter, in the periventricular regions (Figs. 13A, C, and D). The periventricular white matter of the centrum semiovale is of normal signal intensity. There is also a band-like area of white matter signal intensity interposed between the gray matter signal intensity of the cortex and the gray matter signal intensity noted in the periventricular white matter. These signal characteristics are confirmed on the T2-weighted axial images (Figs. 13E–G). The ventricular system and midline structures are otherwise unremarkable (Fig. 13A).

The number of sulci and gyri is slightly decreased with broad flat gyri identified. No other areas of abnormal signal intensity are identified.

Diagnosis

Band (laminar) heterotopia.

Discussion

Gray matter heterotopia is strictly defined as gray matter in an abnormal location. Heterotopia is usually classified as nodular or laminar. The nodular form presents as nodules of gray matter in the subependymal region, typically bilateral. The laminar form presents as areas of gray matter in a linear distribution that may present as holohemispheric gray matter. Band heterotopia, as in this case, presents with diffuse linear gray matter heterotopia. To be classified as band heterotopia there must be white matter signal intensity identified between the cerebral cortical gray matter and the area of heterotopia.

The etiology of gray matter heterotopia is unknown; however, it is thought to relate to events during the time of neuronal migration, e.g., 2–4 months of gestational age. Patients with gray matter heterotopia present with seizures, which sometimes can be intractable, and developmental delay.

The MR features of band heterotopia are as described above and include a layer (or layers) of gray matter signal intensity of variable thickness in the periventricular white matter, separated from the cerebral cortical gray matter by a small amount of periventricular white matter. These patients may have associated pachygyria. Some authors have described the appearance as that of a "three-layered cake."

References

1. Barkovich AJ, Jackson DE Jr, Boyer RS. Band heterotopias: a newly recognized neuronal migration anomaly. *Radiology* 1989;171:455–458.
2. Pollei SR, Boyer RS, Crawford S, et al. Disorders of migration and sulcation. *Semin US CT MR* 1988;9:231–246.

Submitted by: Wayne Davis, M.D., and Richard S. Boyer, M.D., Primary Children's Medical Center, Salt Lake City, Utah; Rosalind B. Dietrich, M.B., Ch.B., Senior Editor.

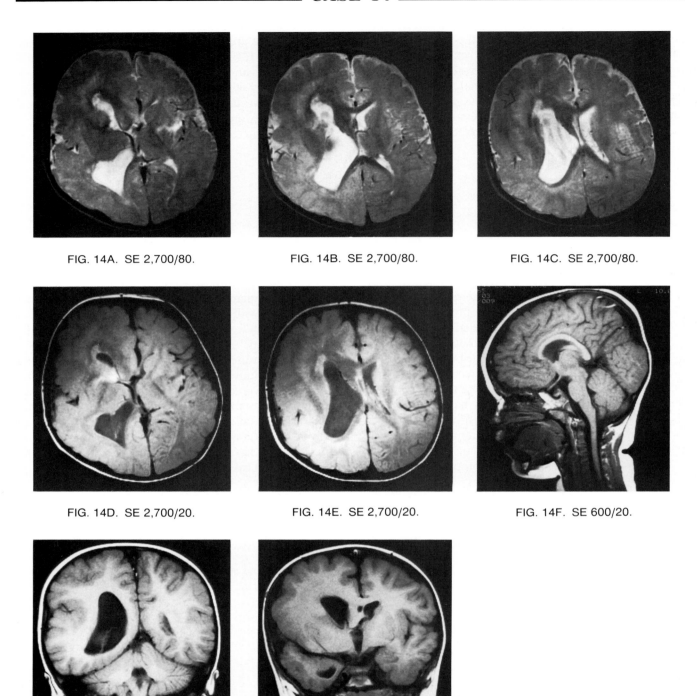

FIG. 14A. SE 2,700/80.

FIG. 14B. SE 2,700/80.

FIG. 14C. SE 2,700/80.

FIG. 14D. SE 2,700/20.

FIG. 14E. SE 2,700/20.

FIG. 14F. SE 600/20.

FIG. 14G. SE 800/20.

FIG. 14H. SE 800/20.

Clinical History

A 19-month-old male with a history of seizures and developmental delay.

Findings

The MR study demonstrates unilateral cerebral hemispheric enlargement with a concomitant shift of the midline. There is ipsilateral ventricular enlargement. On the axial T2-weighted images, abnormal signal intensity is noted in the periventricular white matter regions (Figs. 14A and C, *open arrows*). The sulcation is abnormal with widened gyri and shallow sulci consistent with pachygyria. The gray-white matter interface is ill-defined. There are areas of gray matter signal within the white matter on the T2-weighted images suggestive of heterotopia (Figs. 14B and C, *arrowheads*). The left hemisphere and left lateral ventricle are of normal size and contour. There is mild compression of the right cerebellar hemisphere, which is of otherwise normal signal intensity. The midline structures, including the corpus callosum, are unremarkable.

Diagnosis

Hemimegalencephaly.

Discussion

Hemimegalencephaly is a rare developmental malformation characterized by unilateral hypertrophy of the brain. Its cause is unknown and there is no known familial incidence. Pathologically, giant neurons are diffusely scattered throughout the cortex. Abnormalities of migration and sulcation are frequently identified. Also identified is gliosis within the white matter of the affected cerebral hemisphere.

Patients with hemimegalencephaly typically present with seizures (oftentimes intractable), mental retardation, and macrocephaly or asymmetry of the head shape. In some patients this disorder is lethal in the newborn period. The imaging features of hemimegalencephaly include hypertrophy of one cerebral hemisphere, ipsilateral ventricular enlargement, gyral abnormalities, such as pachygyria, and heterotopia. Areas of T2 hyperintensity are noted within the white matter of the affected cerebral hemisphere. These are thought to be related to the areas of gliosis as described above.

Differential diagnosis includes agyria or pachygyria. These entities can usually be differentiated by their bilaterality and lack of ventricular and white matter signal changes.

References

1. Kalifa GL, Chiron C, Sellier N, et al. Hemimegalencephaly: MR imaging in five children. *Radiology* 1987;165:29–33.
2. Towbin RB, Witte DP, Ball WS Jr, et al. Pediatric case of the day. *Radiographics* 1988;8:573–577.

Submitted by: Wayne Davis, M.D., and Richard S. Boyer, M.D., Primary Children's Medical Center, Salt Lake City, Utah; Rosalind B. Dietrich, M.B., Ch.B., Senior Editor.

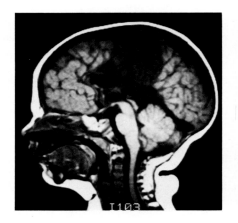

FIG. 15A. SE 500/20.

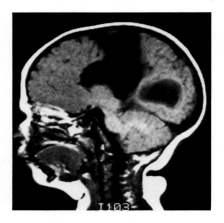

FIG. 15B. SE 500/20.

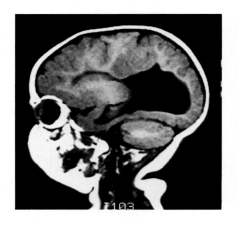

FIG. 15C. SE 500/20.

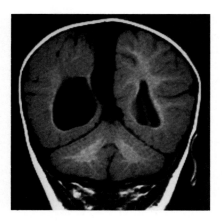

FIG. 15D. SE 800/20.

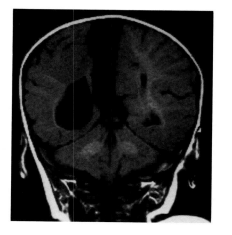

FIG. 15E. SE 800/20.

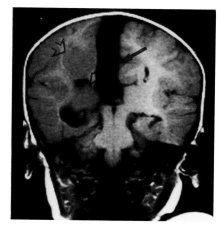

FIG. 15F. SE 800/20.

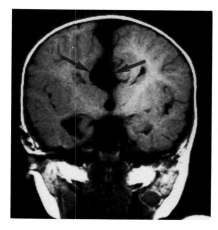

FIG. 15G. SE 800/20.

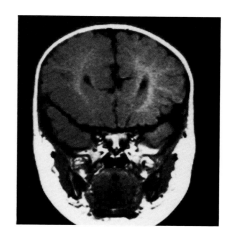

FIG. 15H. SE 800/20.

Clinical History

A 6-month-old white male presented with a history of an abnormal *in utero* ultrasound with suspected intracranial abnormalities. The patient had normal developmental milestones and normal neurologic examination.

Findings

The sagittal T1-weighted sequence demonstrates agenesis of the corpus callosum. There is ventricular enlargement with prominent dilatation of the occipital horns (colpocephaly). Also noted is a CSF-signal intensity cyst in the interhemispheric region extending to the level of the third ventricle and along the right side of the falx cerebrum, most consistent with a dorsal interhemispheric cyst (*arrows*). Gray matter signal intensity is seen in the centrum semiovale of the right parietal lobe in a periventricular location, most consistent with heterotopic gray matter (*arrowheads*).

Diagnosis

Agenesis of the corpus callosum, dorsal interhemispheric cyst, nodular heterotopia.

Discussion

Agenesis of the corpus callosum may present as an isolated lesion (20%) or more commonly in combination with other CNS anomalies (80%). The normal corpus callosum develops between the 12th and 20th weeks of gestation. Dysgenesis is thought to result from insults during the formation of its precursors. Hypoplasia of the corpus callosum is thought to relate to events following formation, i.e., after 20 weeks gestational age. Most cases of agenesis of the corpus callosum are sporadic; however, it has also been associated with chromosomal abnormalities such as trisomy 8 and 13–15D. Patients may present with a variety of clinical features from a normal neurologic exam to seizures and multiple congenital anomalies.

Approximately 80% of cases of agenesis of the corpus callosum are associated with other CNS abnormalities, including interhemispheric cysts (30%), Dandy-Walker malformations and variants (17%), Chiari II malformations, and interhemispheric lipoma. Other less commonly associated abnormalities include cephalocele (nasofrontal and transsphenoidal), septo-optic dysplasia, trigonocephaly, heterotopia, holoprosencephaly, and Aicardia's syndrome.

The MR features of agenesis of the corpus callosum are best evaluated on the midline sagittal T1-weighted sequence where the normally myelinated corpus callosum should be visible. Other features include absence of a portion of the hippocampus or posterior and anterior commissures. The ventricles may demonstrate wide separation and a small size to the frontal horns and enlargement of the occipital horns (colpocephaly). The third ventricle may be enlarged and in a slightly high position. The sagittal T1-weighted sequence may also demonstrate a radial array of the sulci, most prominent in the parietal and parieto-occipital regions due to the lack of formation of the normal pericallosal and cingulate gyri. The coronal T1-weighted sequence may demonstrate collateral callosal bundles, called the bundles of Probst, that form in the medial walls of the bodies and frontal horns of the lateral ventricles. There may be wide separation of the pericallosal arteries and loss of the normal pericallosal sweep and sweep of the internal cerebral vein and

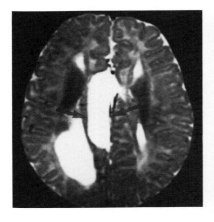

FIG. 15I. SE 4,000/100.

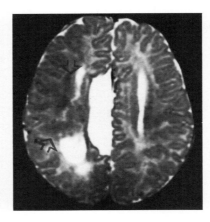

FIG. 15J. SE 4,000/100.

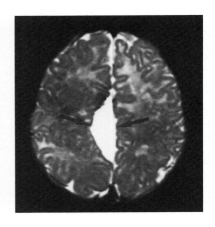

FIG. 15K. SE 4,000/100.

vein of Galen. Additional findings relate to associated CNS abnormalities including the interhemispheric fissure cyst, Dandy-Walker anomalies, and cephaloceles. The lipoma of the corpus callosum is well evaluated with both sagittal and coronal T1-weighted MR by its characteristic high signal intensity. It is stated that agenesis of the corpus callosum is found in 40% of cases of lipoma of the corpus callosum.

References

1. Byrd SE, Osborn RE, Radkowski MA, et al. Disorders of midline structures: holoprosencephaly, absence of corpus callosum, and Chiari malformations. *Semin US CT MR* 1988;9:201–215.
2. Atlas SW, Zimmerman RA, Bilaniuk LT, et al. Corpus callosum and limbic system: neuroanatomic MR evaluation of developmental anomalies. *Radiology* 1986;160:355–352.
3. Barkovich AJ, Kjos BO. Normal postnatal development of the corpus callosum as demonstrated by MR imaging. *AJNR* 1988;9:487–491.
4. Curnes JT, Laster DW, Koubek TD, et al. MRI of corpus callosal syndromes. *AJNR* 1986;7:617–622.
5. Barkovich AJ, Norman D. Anomalies of the corpus callosum: correlation with further anomalies of the brain. *AJNR* 1988;9:493–501.

Submitted by: Wayne Davis, M.D., and Richard S. Boyer, M.D., Primary Children's Medical Center, Salt Lake City, Utah; Rosalind B. Dietrich, M.B., Ch.B., Senior Editor.

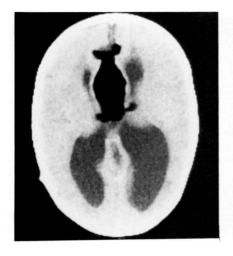

FIG. 16A. CT.

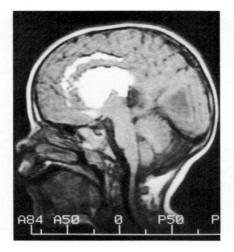

FIG. 16B. SE 600/20.

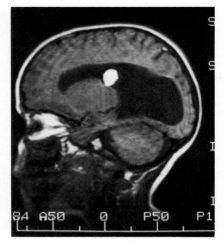

FIG. 16C. SE 600/20.

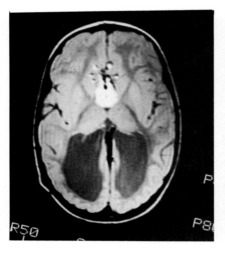

FIG. 16D. SE 2,500/20.

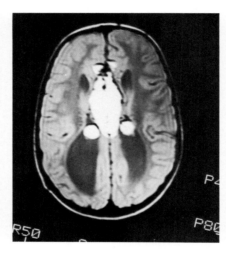

FIG. 16E. SE 2,500/20.

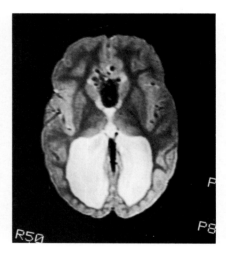

FIG. 16F. SE 2,500/70.

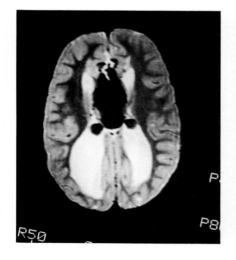

FIG. 16G. SE 2,500/70.

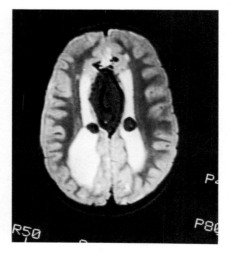

FIG. 16H. SE 2,500/70.

Clinical History

A 5-year-old girl who is mentally retarded with a history of seizures and previous placement of a ventricular shunt.

Findings

CT (Fig. 16A) performed at 1 year of age shows extensive areas of low attenuation in the midline consistent with fat and marked dysplasia of the ventricles. The lateral ventricles appear large, particularly posteriorly.

On MRI, there is seen an extensive area of high signal intensity in the interhemispheric fissure and ventricles on the short TR sequence (Figs. 16B and C) with moderate signal intensity on the T2-weighted images (Fig. 16G). The signal intensities are typical of fat. The gyri of the medial surface of the hemispheres radiate toward the interhemispheric fissure on the midline sagittal image (Fig. 16B), which in this case, as noted, is occupied by fat. The corpus callosum is absent, as seen on the sagittal scan and the axial images (Figs. 16D–H).

The fat surrounds interhemispheric vessels, which are delineated by signal void (Fig. 16G, H) and also extends into the region of the choroid plexus (Fig. 16F).

The atria and occipital horns are large (colpoceptualy), as the splenium is absent. The basal ganglia are more widely separated than normally seen, with CSF occupying the area between them, with low signal intensity on the T1-weighted image (Fig. 16D) and high signal intensity on the T2-weighted image (Fig. 16F). This represents a high and prominent third ventricle. The fat anterior to this lies in the region of the fornix (Fig. 16D).

No heterotopic gray matter is identified.

Diagnosis

Lipoma of the corpus callosum with callosal agenesis.

Discussion

Lipoma of the corpus callosum is a congenital malformation of the brain, best classified with the midline dysraphias (1). It is a disorder of cerebral hemispheric organization (1). The interhemispheric collections of primitive and mature fat lie in or near the corpus callosum. Lipomas may be asymptomatic but more commonly present with seizures, mental disturbances, paralysis, or headache (1).

On MRI, a midline collection of fat is seen, hyperintense on T1-weighted sequences, in the interhemispheric fissure, usually near the genu of the corpus callosum. There may be extension around the splenium, through the choroidal fissure, along cerebral clefts, and through a cranium bifidum (1).

Encasement of interhemispheric arteries by the fat can occur, with fusiform dilatation of the vessel sometimes seen. There is also an increased incidence of anomalous anterior cerebral arteries (1).

In as many as 50% of patients with lipomas there is also callosal dysgenesis, as seen in this case.

Retrocerebellar arachnoid cysts, Dandy-Walker cyst, and Dandy-Walker variant as a group occur with an increased incidence in agenesis of the corpus callosum (2).

Incidence of intracranial lipomas at autopsy is slightly less than 0.1%. In addition to the midline location, they may also be seen at the quadrigeminal plate tuber cinereum and cerebellopontine angles. Small lipomas are not infrequently seen on MRI as incidental findings in asymptomatic patients and are clearly identifiable by their signal intensities as discussed.

References

1. Naidich TP, Zimmerman RA. Common congenital malformations of the brain. In: Brant-Zawadski M, Norman D, eds. *Magnetic resonance imaging of the central nervous system.* New York: Raven Press, 1987;131–151.
2. Byrd SE, Naidich TP. Common congenital brain anomalies. *Radiol Clin North Am* 1988;26:755–770.

Submitted by: Patricia E. Perry, M.D., Good Samaritan Regional Medical Center and Phoenix Children's Hospital, Phoenix, Arizona; Rosalind B. Dietrich, M.B., Ch.B., Senior Editor.

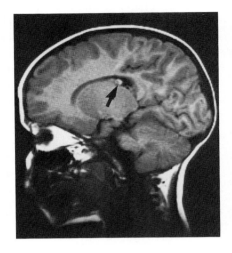

FIG. 17A. SE 500/20.

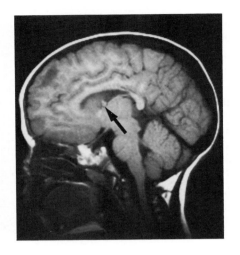

FIG. 17B. SE 500/20.

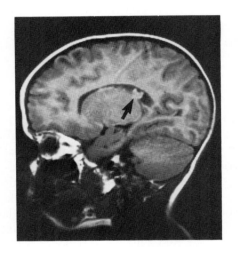

FIG. 17C. SE 500/20.

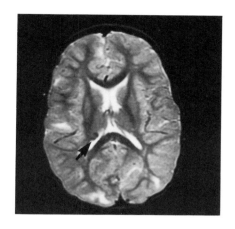

FIG. 17D. SE 2,500/80.

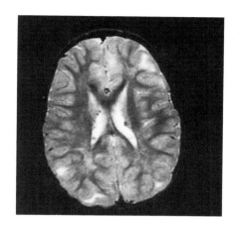

FIG. 17E. SE 2,500/80.

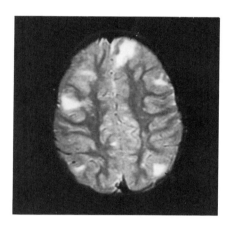

FIG. 17F. SE 2,500/80.

Clinical History

A $2\frac{1}{2}$-year-old male with a seizure disorder.

Findings

The sagittal T1-weighted MR sequence demonstrates areas of intermediate signal intensity in the subependymal region of the lateral ventricles (Figs. 17A–C, *arrows*). On the axial and coronal T2-weighted images, these areas of signal abnormality vary from intermittent to very low signal intensity (Figs. 17D, G–I, *arrows*). A CT scan was also performed that demonstrated periventricular calcification in locations corresponding to very low signal intensity seen on these T2-weighted images. Multiple areas of T2 hyperintensity are identified scattered throughout the cerebral cortex (Figs. 17E, F, H, and I, *arrowheads*). Also noted are areas of T2 hyperintensity in the peritrigonal cerebral white matter seen on both the coronal and axial T2-weighted images. The midline structures and ventricles are within normal limits.

Diagnosis

Tuberous sclerosis.

Discussion

Tuberous sclerosis is an autosomal dominant disorder with a high incidence of spontaneous mutations. Hamartomatous lesions are seen in the CNS, heart, kidney, skeletal, and lungs.

The classic clinical triad is adenoma sebaceum, mental retardation, and seizures. These three clinical features are seen only in a portion of the patients with tuberous sclerosis. Other cutaneous manifestations include shagreen patches, subungual fibromas, and café-au-lait spots. Retinal phakomas are seen in a high percentage of patients.

The CNS manifestations of tuberous sclerosis consist of hamartomas, which are present in the subependymal and cortical regions of both hemispheres. The term "tuber" comes from the gross pathologic description by Bourneville of the cortical hamartomas. Giant cell astrocytomas occur in tuberous sclerosis, and these are thought to be secondary to degeneration within one of the subependymal nodules. It is estimated that giant cell astrocytomas occur in 5%–15% of patients with tuberous sclerosis.

Patients with tuberous sclerosis also develop areas of demyelination within the periventricular white matter. Nonobstructive dilatation of the ventricular system has been identified in tuberous sclerosis, as seen in some patients with neurofibromatosis.

The MR appearance of tuberous sclerosis is characteristic with intermediate T1 signal intensity nodules seen in the subependymal regions of the lateral ventricles. They are rarely seen about the third or fourth ventricle. A few of these may contain very low signal intensity corresponding to calcium seen typically on CT. The cortical hamartomas present as areas of ill-defined T2 hyperintensity. Gyral enlargement is seen in the areas of cortical hamartoma formation. MR is far more sensitive for the detection of cortical hamartomas as compared to CT. An additional finding on MR are areas of T2 hyperintensity within the cerebral white matter that relate to

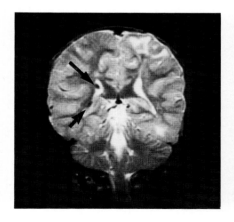

FIG. 17G. SE 2,500/80.

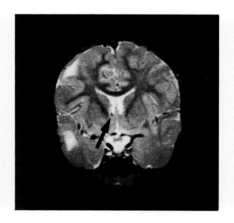

FIG. 17H. SE 2,500/80.

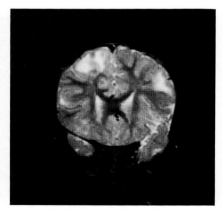

FIG. 17I. SE 2,500/80.

areas of demyelination and/or white matter hamartomatous lesions. Giant cell astrocytomas are typically detected on CT by demonstration of contrast enhancement of a subependymal nodule. These lesions are frequently located in the region of the foramen of Monro. Although there are reports in the MR literature of a development of T2 hyperintensity and enhancement following administration of gadolinium-DTPA in giant cell astrocytomas, further investigation is needed to confirm MR's applicability in this area.

In addition to CNS imaging, patients with tuberous sclerosis need to undergo echocardiography and renal sonography to exclude rhabdomyomas and angiomyolipomas.

References

1. Crawford SC, Boyer RS, Harnsberger HR, et al. Disorders of histogenesis: the neurocutaneous syndromes. *Sem in US CT MR* 1988;9:247–267.
2. McMurdo SK Jr, Moore SG, Brant-Zawadzki M, et al. MR imaging of intracranial tuberous sclerosis. *AJNR* 1987;8:77–82.
3. Braffman BH, Bilaniuk LT, Zimmerman RA. The central nervous system manifestations of the phakomatoses on MR. *Radiol Clin North Am* 1988;26:773–796.

Submitted by: Wayne Davis, M.D., and Richard S. Boyer, M.D., Primary Children's Medical Center, Salt Lake City, Utah; Rosalind B. Dietrich, M.B., Ch.B., Senior Editor.

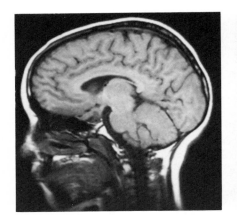

FIG. 18A. SE 600/20.

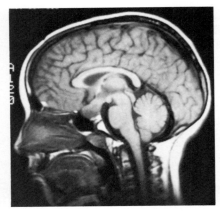

FIG. 18B. SE 600/20.

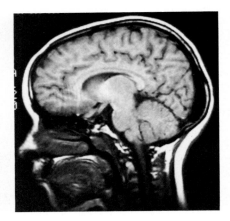

FIG. 18C. SE 600/20.

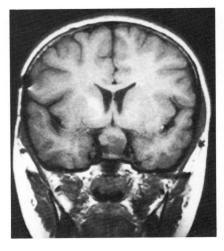

FIG. 18D. SE 600/20.

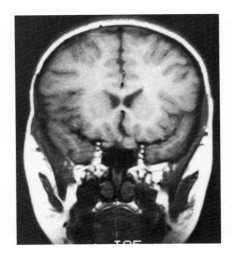

FIG. 18E. SE 600/20.

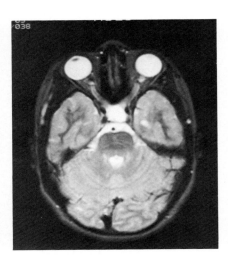

FIG. 18F. SE 2,500/80.

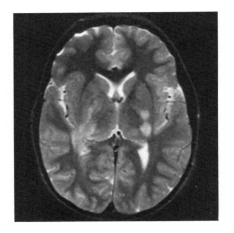

FIG. 18G. SE 2,500/80.

Clinical History

An 8-year-old female with café-au-lait spots and decreased vision who 3 years previously was diagnosed to have a brain tumor.

Findings

An MR study performed on 9/2/87 (Figs. 18A–G) demonstrated enlarged optic nerves and chiasm with mixed signal in the distribution of the optic radiations and tracts. There are patchy areas of bright signal on T1-weighted, proton density, and heavily T2-weighted scans.

A follow-up study on 8/17/88 demonstrated similar findings. After gadolinium injection, T1-weighted images show bright enhancement in the region of the optic chiasm but no enhancement of the retrochiasmatic portion of the tumor (Figs. 18H and I).

Diagnosis

Neurofibromatosis 1 with optic pathway glioma.

Discussion

Neurofibromatosis (von Recklinghausen's disease) is an inherited neurocutaneous disorder with autosomal dominance with variable penetrance and a high spontaneous mutation rate. It is characterized by cutaneous pigmentation and multiple tumors originating from neuroectodermal elements. Manifestations are protean and may involve any organ system. Skin manifestations include café-au-lait spots and molluscum fibrosum. Endocrine abnormalities include pheochromocytoma. CNS involvement includes cerebral cortical underdevelopment, neoplasms, hydrocephalus, arachnoid cysts, psammomatous calcifications, hydrosyringomyelia, neurofibromas, meningiomas, and spinal cord gliomas. Skeletal abnormalities involve the skull, spine, and long bones. Respiratory, gastrointestinal, genitourinary, and cardiovascular lesions are also seen.

There are two genetically separate types of neurofibromatosis. Neurofibromatosis 1 is the classic von Recklinghausen's disease, which is associated with CNS tumors of astrocytes and neurons. It presents at a younger age and its intracranial manifestations include optic gliomas, astrocytomas, "hamartomas," and neurofibromas. Neurofibromatosis 2 is associated with bilateral acoustic neuromas and meningiomas. The intracranial manifestations are limited to schwannomas and meningiomas. Criteria for differentiating the two types are published.

MR findings relate to the site of CNS tumors and include optic nerve and pathway gliomas, acoustic neuromas, meningiomas, gliomas outside the optic pathway, cerebral hamartomas, plexiform neurofibromas of peripheral nerves, buphthalmos, dysplasia of the greater wing of the sphenoid, calvarial defects, and cerebral arterial occlusive disease.

References

1. Aoki S, Barkovich AJ, Nishimura K, et al. Neurofibromatosis types 1 and 2: cranial MR findings. *Radiology* 1989;172:527–534.
2. Crawford SC, Boyer RH, Harnsberger HR, et al. Disorders of histogenesis: the neurocutaneous syndromes. *Semin US CT MR* 1988;9:247–267.

Submitted by: Arthur Watanabe, M.D., and Richard S. Boyer, M.D., Primary Children's Medical Center, Salt Lake City, Utah; Rosalind B. Dietrich, M.B., Ch.B., Senior Editor.

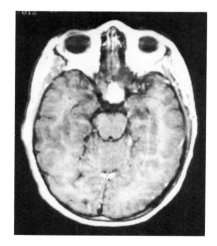

FIG. 18H. SE 500/20 with Gd-DTPA.

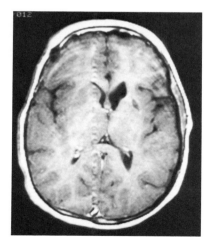

FIG. 18I. SE 500/20 with Gd-DTPA.

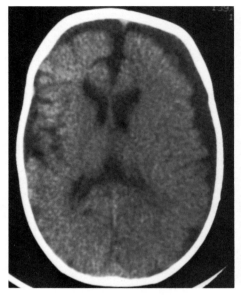

FIG. 19A. CT. At 2 months of age.

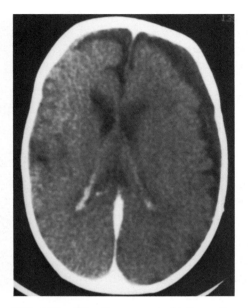

FIG. 19B. CT with contrast. At 2 months of age.

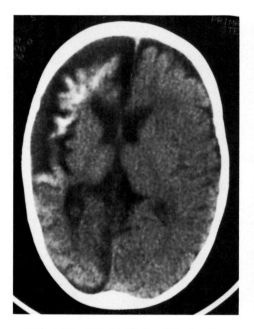

FIG. 19C. CT. At 12 months of age.

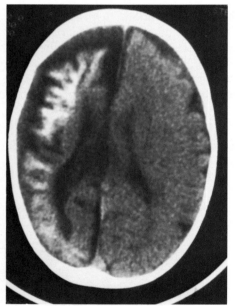

FIG. 19D. CT. At 12 months of age.

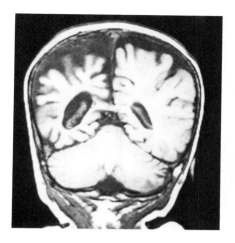
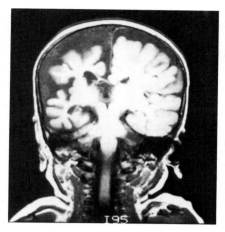
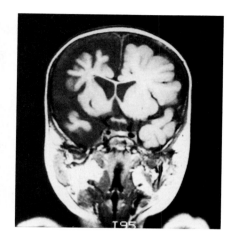

FIG. 19E. SE 800/20.   FIG. 19F. SE 800/20.   FIG. 19G. SE 800/20.

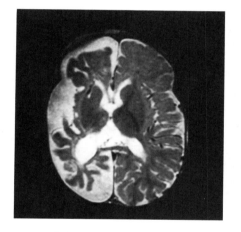
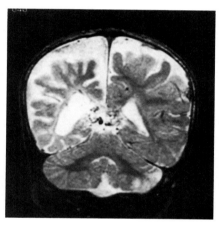
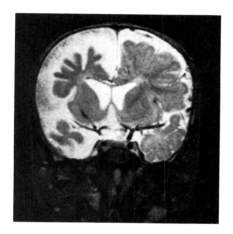

FIG. 19H. SE 3,000/80.   FIG. 19I. SE 3,000/80.   FIG. 19J. SE 3,000/80.

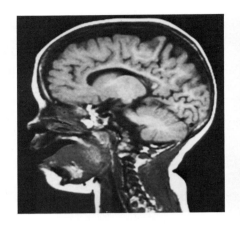

FIG. 19K. SE 600/20.

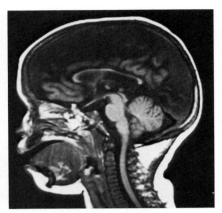

FIG. 19L. SE 600/20.

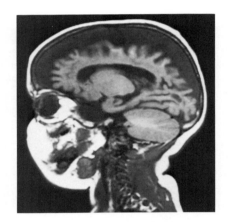

FIG. 19M. SE 600/20.

Clinical History

A child with a port-wine stain on the right side of the face presented at 2 months with seizures.

44

Findings

Copies of the CT studies when the child was 2 (Figs. 19A and B) and 12 (Figs. 19C and D) months of age are submitted. The initial study was performed before and after contrast injection. On the pre-contrast study, faint increased attenuation in the right hemisphere indicates early calcification and mild atrophy (Fig. 19A). No abnormal enhancement is seen in the hemisphere. The choroid plexus is mildly prominent on the right. A follow-up CT scan 10 months later demonstrates progressive atrophy and calcification of the right cerebral hemisphere (Fig. 19C and D).

Multiplanar brain MR demonstrates right-sided cerebral hemiatrophy with ipsilateral enlargement of the extraaxial CSF spaces and lateral ventricle (Figs. 19E–J). No calcification is identified. Unfortunately, this study was performed before MR contrast became routinely available; therefore, we cannot comment on the enhancing characteristics of the lesion from the MR study.

Diagnosis

Sturge-Weber syndrome.

Discussion

Sturge-Weber syndrome, also known as encephalotrigeminal angiomatosis, is a congenital disorder of unknown etiology characterized by a facial port-wine nevus along the distribution of the trigeminal nerve with ipsilateral leptomeningeal angiomatosis and subjacent cerebral hemisphere atrophy with intracortical calcifications. It is usually unilateral but may be bilateral. Ocular involvement may manifest as buphthalmos or choroid angiomas. Epilepsy, mental retardation, limb atrophy contralateral to facial nevus, and hemisensory deficit are common.

MR findings include atrophy of one hemisphere, especially in occipital and temporal lobes, with shrunken calcified gyri and enlarged sulci; superficial leptomeningeal angiomas; and nonfunctional or absent cortical veins with patent deep veins. With contrast, there may be diffuse enhancement of the affected hemisphere with a prominently enhancing ipsilateral choroid plexus due to the deep venous drainage.

Reference

1. Crawford SC, Boyer RS, Harnsberger HR, et al. Disorders of histogenesis: the neurocutaneous syndromes. *Semin US CT MR* 1988;9:247–267.

Submitted by: Arthur Watanabe, M.D., and Richard S. Boyer, M.D., Primary Children's Medical Center, Salt Lake City, Utah; Rosalind B. Dietrich, M.B., Ch.B., Senior Editor.

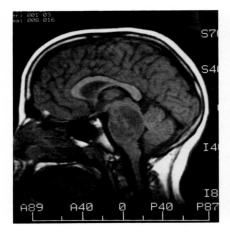

FIG. 20A. SE 600/20.

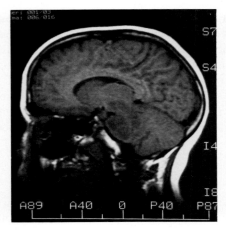

FIG. 20B. SE 600/20.

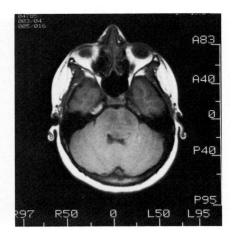

FIG. 20C. SE 600/20.

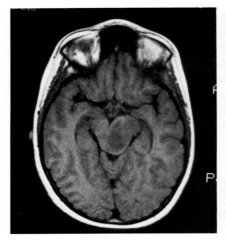

FIG. 20D. SE 600/20.

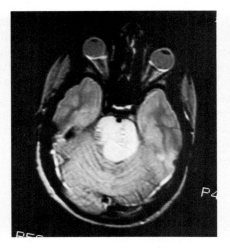

FIG. 20E. SE 2,500/45.

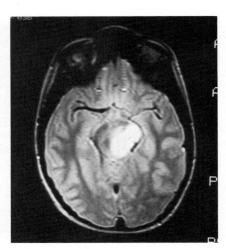

FIG. 20F. SE 2,500/45.

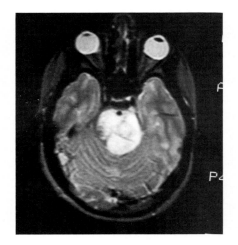

FIG. 20G. SE 2,500/90.

Clinical History

A 12-year-old male presented with difficulty swallowing and gait disturbance.

46

Findings

There is marked enlargement of the pons and left side of the midbrain. The involved areas demonstrate heterogeneous decreased signal intensity on T1-weighted images and increased signal intensity on intermediate- and T2-weighted images. The fourth ventricle is compressed. There is no evidence of hydrocephalus.

Diagnosis

Brain stem glioma.

Discussion

Brain stem gliomas are common in the pediatric age group, accounting for 10%–25% of all intracranial tumors in childhood (1).

The clinical presentation usually consists of multiple bilateral cranial nerve dysfunction and varying degrees of motor dysfunction in the arms and/or legs (2).

The site most frequently involved is the pons, followed by the midbrain and then medulla. Exophytic growth may also occur in the prepontine and cerebellopontine angle cisterns. The tumors may also grow longitudinally to involve the entire brain stem and extend into the upper cervical cord. The majority of the lesions are highly malignant (3). Pathologically these tumors may demonstrate cyst formation, necrosis, and hemorrhage.

On MRI these tumors typically demonstrate enlargement of the pons with associated compression of the fourth ventricle.

Hydrocephalus is usually a late finding. The tumors are predominantly decreased signal intensity on T1-weighted images and increased signal intensity on T2-weighted images. Cystic or necrotic areas are usually higher signal intensity on T2-weighted images than the adjacent solid tumor. Enhancement following gadolinium-DTPA administration is similar to that observed on post-contrast CT, varying from none to diffuse. The degree of enhancement does not correlate with the degree of malignancy or exact tumor margins (4).

References

1. Stroink AR, Hoffman HJ, Hendrick EB, Humphreys RP. Diagnosis and management of pediatric brain-stem gliomas. *J Neurosurg* 1986;65:745–750.
2. Albright AL, Guthkelch AN, Packer RJ, Price RA, Rourke LB. Prognostic factors in pediatric brain-stem gliomas. *J Neurosurg* 1986;65:751–755.
3. Epstein F, McCleary EL. Intrinsic brain-stem tumors of childhood: surgical indications. *J Neurosurg* 1986;64:11–15.
4. Tsuchida T, Shimbo Y, Fukuda M, Takeda N, Tanaka R, Ikuta F. Computed tomographic and histopathological studies of pontine glioma. *Childs Nerv Syst* 1985;1:223–229.

Submitted by: C. Roger Bird, M.D., Barrow Neurological Institute, Phoenix, Arizona; Rosalind B. Dietrich, M.B., Ch.B., Senior Editor.

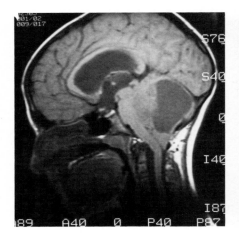

FIG. 21A. SE 600/20.

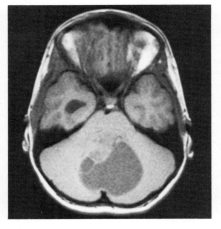

FIG. 21B. SE 600/20.

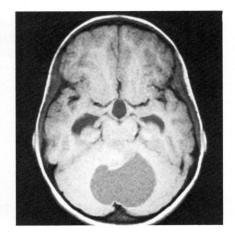

FIG. 21C. SE 600/20.

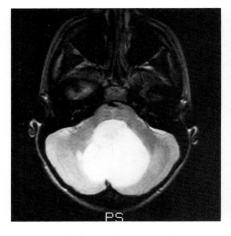

FIG. 21D. SE 2,500/40.

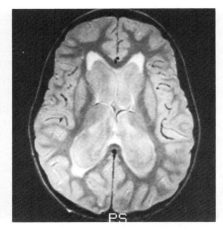

FIG. 21E. SE 2,500/40.

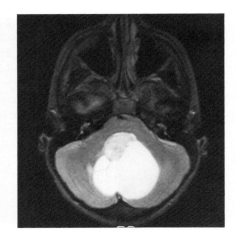

FIG. 21F. SE 2,500/80.

Clinical History

An 8-year-old boy with headaches.

Findings

Large mass arising in the cerebellar vermis and extending into the cerebellar hemispheres. The majority of the mass appears cystic, having well-defined margins with homogeneous low signal on T1-weighted images and high signal on intermediate- and T2-weighted images. The anterior portion of the mass appears more solid with heterogeneous signal characteristics. There is compression of the posterior brain stem. There is moderate obstructive hydrocephalus due to compression of the fourth ventricle. Periventricular hyperintensity is consistent with transependymal edema.

Diagnosis

Cerebellar astrocytoma.

Discussion

Cerebellar astrocytoma is predominantly a tumor of childhood and has the most favorable overall prognosis of all childhood brain tumors. Most are of the very benign "juvenile pilocytic" histologic type. Cerebellar glioblastoma is a rare but highly malignant tumor with a propensity for leptomeningeal spread (1).

Cerebellar astrocytomas are usually seen in the first two decades of life and have a peak incidence at approximately 7 years of age (2). They occur with equal frequency in males and females. The clinical presentation may include headache, vomiting, and cerebellar signs such as truncal ataxia or dysdiadochokinesia. Cerebellar astrocytomas may originate near the midline or in the hemisphere, and some authors report a slight predominance of tumors in the hemispheres (3). Cystic astrocytomas with mural nodules represent approximately 50% of all cerebellar astrocytomas. Another 40%–45% have a solid rim and a cystic or necrotic center. Less than 10% are nonnecrotic solid tumors, although the solid tumors have a somewhat less favorable prognosis (1).

On MRI, cerebellar astrocytoma is typically a large, circumscribed, predominantly cystic vermian or hemispheric mass. The tumor is generally hypointense on T1-weighted images and hyperintense on T2-weighted images. Solid portions of the tumor are usually heterogeneous; occasionally the solid component is homogeneous and may simulate a cyst. Contrast enhancement is often irregular but almost always present. Hydrocephalus is common, due to compression of the fourth ventricle. Extension of tumor into the brain stem or spinal cord may also be seen. Calcification has been noted histologically in 20% of cerebellar astrocytomas and may be seen on CT or MRI (1). Tumor hemorrhage is rare.

The differential diagnosis includes medulloblastoma and ependymoma. However, although these two tumors tend to fill and dilate the fourth ventricle, cerebellar astrocytomas often extrinsically compress the fourth ventricle. Moreover, the macrocysts commonly seen in cerebellar astrocytoma rarely occur in medulloblastoma or ependymoma (2).

References

1. Barkovich AJ. *Pediatric neuroimaging.* New York: Raven Press, 1990;150–151.
2. Lee Y-Y, Tassel PV, Bruner JM, Moser RP, Share JC. Juvenile pilocytic astrocytomas: CT and MR characteristics. *AJNR* 1989;10:363–370.
3. Russell DS, Rubenstein LJ. *Pathology of tumors of the nervous system,* 5th ed. Baltimore: Williams and Wilkins, 1989;152–159.

Submitted by: David F. Winfield, M.D., Barrow Neurological Institute, Phoenix, Arizona; Rosalind B. Dietrich, M.B., Ch.B., Senior Editor.

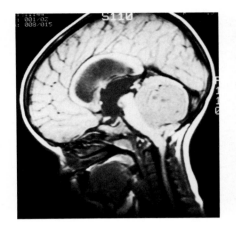

FIG. 22A. SE 800/20.

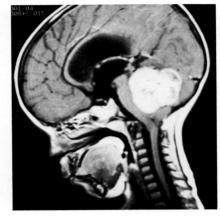

FIG. 22B. SE 700/16.

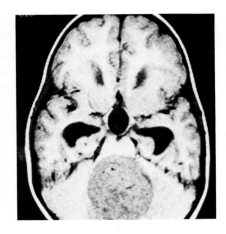

FIG. 22C. SE 800/20.

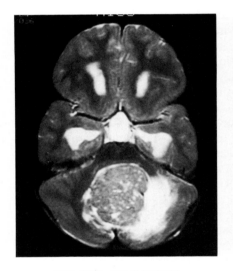

FIG. 22D. SE 2,800/90.

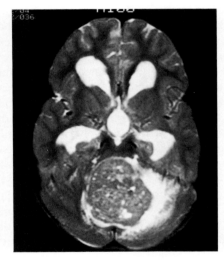

FIG. 22E. SE 2,800/90.

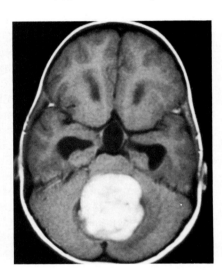

FIG. 22F. SE 750/16 with Gd-DTPA.

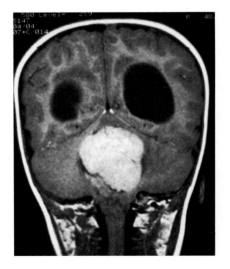

FIG. 22G. SE 400/20 with Gd-DTPA.

Clinical History

A 2-year-old female with sudden onset of vomiting, headache, and severe ataxia.

Findings

An approximately 5 cm midline posterior fossa mass is filling or compressing the fourth ventricle. The mass enhances intensely with gadolinium. Marked bilateral periventricular high signal intensity is noted compatible with transependymal migration of CSF with a marked degree of hydrocephalus.

Diagnosis

Medulloblastoma.

Discussion

Medulloblastomas comprise approximately 7%–8% of all intracranial tumors of neuroepithelial origin, 25% of intracranial tumors in children; 50% occur in the first decade (1). They usually arise in the cerebellum, classically in the midline behind the fourth ventricle, compressing as well as extending into the fourth ventricle. Less commonly, medulloblastoma may be found laterally in the cerebellar hemispheres. The incidence of subarachnoid cerebrospinal metastases is approximately 10%–15% (2).

Medulloblastoma originates from the fetal granular layer (1). Histologically, the tumor is composed of densely crowded dark-staining cells and is usually well circumscribed grossly. Central necrosis is seen only in very large lesions and calcification is uncommon. The classic MRI appearance is that of a homogeneous, well-circumscribed, intensely enhancing lesion with long T1 and T2 relaxation times (3).

Differential considerations include ependymoma (arising from the ependymal lining of the ventricles and frequently calcified) as well as cerebellar astrocytoma (characteristically arising from cerebellar hemispheres or vermis).

References

1. Russell DS, Rubinstein LJ. *Pathology of tumors of the nervous system,* 5th ed. Baltimore: Williams and Wilkins, 1989;251–279.
2. Okazaki H. *Fundamentals of neuropathology.* New York, Tokyo: Igaku-Shoin, 1983;202–207.
3. Brant-Zawadzki M, Norman D. *Magnetic resonance imaging of the central nervous system.* New York: Raven Press, 1987;179–185.

Submitted by: Eric C. Flint, M.D., and C. Roger Bird, M.D., Barrow Neurological Institute, Phoenix, Arizona; Rosalind B. Dietrich, M.B., Ch.B., Senior Editor.

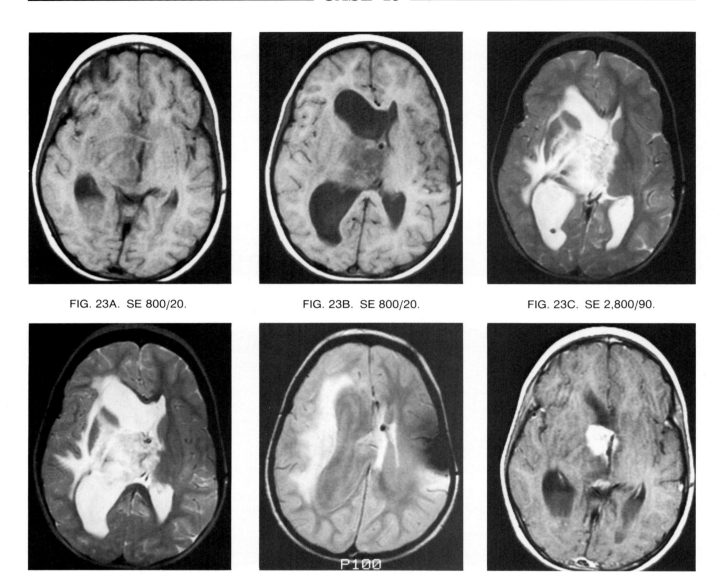

FIG. 23A. SE 800/20.

FIG. 23B. SE 800/20.

FIG. 23C. SE 2,800/90.

FIG. 23D. SE 2,800/90.

FIG. 23E. SE 2,800/30.

FIG. 23F. SE 800/20 with Gd-DTPA.

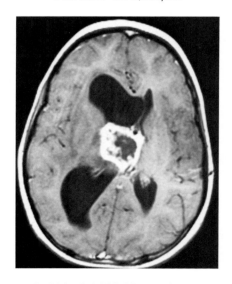

FIG. 23G. SE 800/20 with Gd-DTPA.

Clinical History

A previously healthy 7-year-old female presented with progressive nausea and headache.

Findings

An irregular 4.5 cm rim enhancing mass noted in the right thalamus. The margins of enhancement extend across midline into the third ventricle and the body of the left lateral ventricle. There is a central hypointense portion on T1-weighted images consistent with necrosis. Extensive white matter hyperintensity on intermediate- and T2-weighted images surrounds the mass and extends into the deep white matter tracts of the right cerebral hemisphere, superiorly into the right corona radiata and centrum semiovale, and inferiorly into the midbrain, where it also crosses the midline to the left side. There is hydrocephalus and metallic artifact in the left parietal region from a shunt catheter.

Diagnosis

Glioblastoma multiforme (GBM) of the right thalamus with subependymal spread around the third ventricle.

Discussion

Gliomas arise from the native glial elements of the brain. GBM is a term reserved for a classification of glioma with abundant glial pleomorphism, numerous mitotic figures and giant cells, pseudopalisading of cells, and vascular hyperplasia. They constitute at least 60% of all gliomas and occur most commonly in a supratentorial white matter location, during middle age, and more commonly in men than women (1). Because they are rapidly growing, presenting symptoms are often secondary to increased intracranial pressure (headache, nausea) or local invasion (focal neurologic deficits) (2). GBM has a white matter preference of spread and may extend across the midline through structures such as corpus callosum (butterfly glioma) (3).

On T2-weighted MR images, GBMs appear as irregular, high signal intensity lesions with surrounding edema. Tumor cells may extend into these areas of edema (4). Signal heterogeneity may reflect necrosis, cyst formation, and/or calcification; this glioma is termed "multiforme." The central tumor may often be distinguished from surrounding edema by the edema's shorter T1 and longer T2 relaxation times. However, distinction between tumor and edema may be more consistently shown with administration of contrast material such as gadolinium-DTPA. Multifocal tumor is identified in approximately 5% of cases, and if the GBM reaches the ventricular surface of cortical gyri, seeding via the CSF is common.

Principal differential diagnoses include a single metastatic lesion or abscess.

References

1. Stark DD, Bradley WG. *Magnetic resonance imaging.* St. Louis: C. V. Mosby, 1988.
2. Ramsey RG. *Neuroradiology,* 2nd ed. Philadelphia: W. B. Saunders, 1987.
3. Russell DS, Rubinstein LJ. *Pathology of tumors of the nervous system,* 4th ed. Baltimore: Williams and Wilkins, 1977.
4. Johnson PC, Hunt SJ, Drayer BP. Human cerebral gliomas: correlation of postmortem MR imaging and neuropathologic findings. *Radiology* 1989;170:211.

Submitted by: Tom Knight, M.D., and C. Roger Bird, M.D., Barrow Neurological Institute, Phoenix, Arizona; Rosalind B. Dietrich, M.B., Ch.B., Senior Editor.

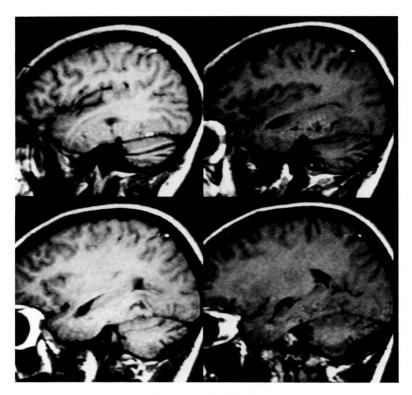

FIG. 24A. SE 600/20.

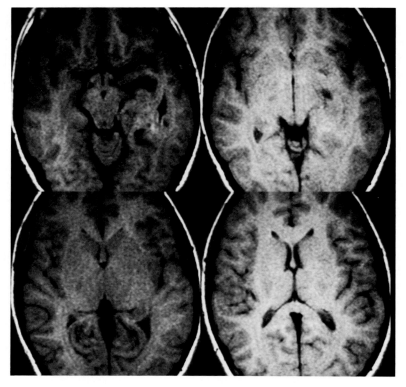

FIG. 24B. SE 800/20.

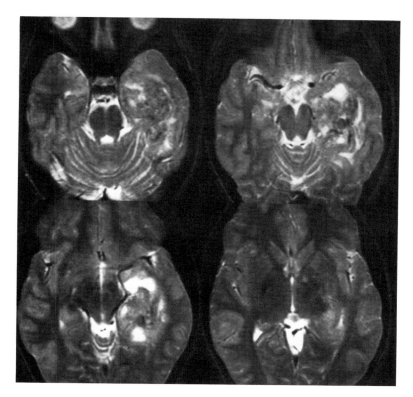

FIG. 24C. SE 2,500/90.

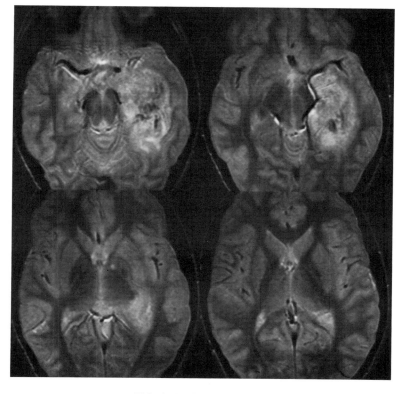

FIG. 24D. SE 2,500/30.

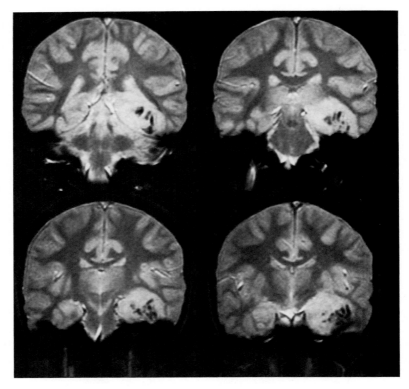

FIG. 24E. SE 2,500/30.

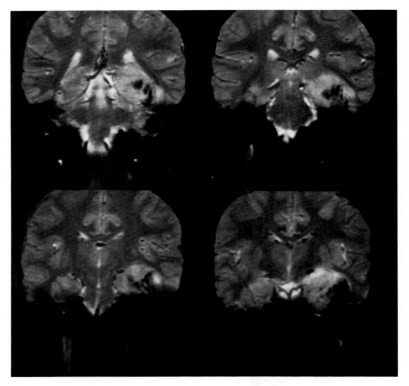

FIG. 24F. GRE 750/15/20°.

Clinical History

A 12-year-old male with seizures.

Findings

Left temporal lobe mass with heterogeneous isointense-hypointense signal intensity on T1-weighted images (Figs. 24A and B), and mixed increased and decreased signal on T2-weighted images (Fig. 24C). Foci of marked hypointensity on gradient-echo coronal sequences (Figs. 24E and F) likely represent calcification. There is mild dilatation of the left temporal horn.

Diagnosis

Ganglioglioma.

Discussion

Ganglioglioma is a slow-growing, usually benign tumor of the CNS. Histologically, the tumor is composed of mature ganglion cells and supporting stromal elements derived from glial tissue; ganglioneuroma is a closely related tumor in which neuronal, rather than glial, elements predominate (1).

Ganglioglioma occurs in all age groups, but most commonly in children and young adults; approximately 60% occur in patients under 30 years of age (2). The clinical presentation usually includes long-standing or worsening headaches or seizures. Gangliogliomas occur most frequently in the cerebral hemispheres, especially in the temporal lobe; the third ventricle, hypothalamus, cerebellum, brain stem, and spinal cord may also be affected. Gangliogliomas are usually single but may occasionally be multiple (3).

On MRI, the ganglioglioma is usually a well-circumscribed lesion of mixed signal intensity on T1-weighted sequences and high signal intensity on T2-weighted sequences; foci of increased signal on T1-weighted images may be characteristic (1). Mass effect is usually minimal. The tumor is usually peripherally located within the hemispheres and erosion of the overlying calvarium may be seen. Cystic components may be present, and CT has demonstrated calcification in approximately 35% of gangliogliomas (2). Contrast enhancement is variable and may be completely absent.

The differential diagnosis includes astrocytoma and oligodendroglioma when the tumor is located peripherally, and hypothalamic glioma when located in the hypothalamic region.

References

1. Barkovich AJ. *Pediatric neuroimaging.* New York: Raven Press, 1990;182–183.
2. Dorne HL, O'Gorman AM, Melanson D. Computed tomography of intracranial gangliogliomas. *AJNR* 1986;7:281–285.
3. Russell DS, Rubenstein LJ. *Pathology of tumors of the nervous system,* 5th ed. Baltimore: Williams and Wilkins, 1989;289–306.

Submitted by: David F. Winfield, M.D., and C. Roger Bird, M.D., Barrow Neurological Institute, Phoenix, Arizona; Rosalind B. Dietrich, M.B., Ch.B., Senior Editor.

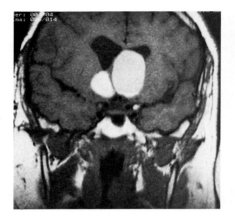

FIG. 25A. SE 600/20.

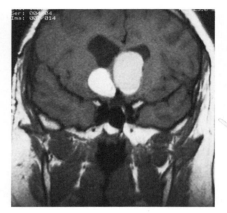

FIG. 25B. SE 600/20.

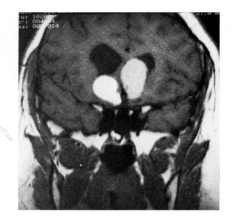

FIG. 25C. SE 600/20.

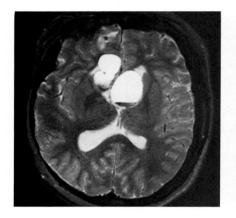

FIG. 25D. SE 2,800/90.

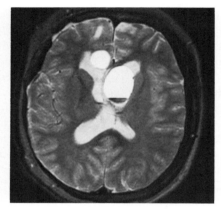

FIG. 25E. SE 2,800/90.

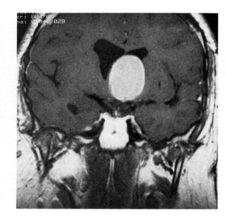

FIG. 25F. SE 600/20 with Gd-DTPA.

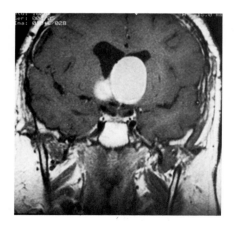

FIG. 25G. SE 600/20 with Gd-DTPA.

Clinical History

A 14-year-old female with worsening vision and pituitary dysfunction.

Findings

A large multilobulated mass projects superiorly from the suprasellar region with impression upon the hypothalamic/thalamic regions; this mass demonstrates increased signal intensity on T1- and T2-weighted images, with a fluid level of decreased signal layering posteriorly on T2-weighted axial images. The largest component shows definite rim enhancement. There is evidence of obstruction at the level of the foramen of Monro with dilatation of the lateral ventricles.

Diagnosis

Craniopharyngioma.

Discussion

Craniopharyngioma represents one of the most common supratentorial tumors of childhood. Approximately one-half of cases present during the first and second decades, with a second peak during the fifth decade (1). These tumors are benign, slow-growing, and well-defined suprasellar masses that usually present with headache, visual complaints, and symptoms caused by dysfunction of the hypothalamus and pituitary gland, including growth failure (2). Histologically, craniopharyngiomas are composed of nests or trabeculae of epithelial cells and/or epithelial-lined cysts embedded in a loose connective tissue glial stroma. Cells may be arranged in solid nests of squamous cells or in an adamantanomatous pattern. Grossly, they may be either largely cystic, containing straw-colored, thick fluid rich in cholesterol or partially cystic and solid (1). Approximately 75% contain calcium.

The pathologic variability is reflected in their MR appearance. High intensity on T1-weighted images has been demonstrated within cystic lesions containing high lipid content or methemoglobin. Moderate intensity on T1-weighted images has been demonstrated in tumors lacking significant lipid or hemorrhage. Both groups demonstrate high signal intensity on T2-weighted images (2).

The origin of such lesions remains unsettled (1). Possible etiologies include

A. Squamous cell nests, remnants of Rathke's pouch, at the junction of the pituitary infundibulum and the pars distalis,
B. Midline congenital tumor not fundamentally different from an epidermoid cyst,
C. Inclusion of the dental anlage, identical to adamantanoma of the jaw.

References

1. Okazaki H. *Fundamentals of neuropathology.* New York, Tokyo: Igaku-Shoin, 1983.
2. Pusey E, Kortman KE, Flannigan BD. MR of craniopharyngiomas: tumor delineation and characterization. *AJNR* 1987;8:439–444.
3. Petito CK, DeGirolami U, Earle KM. Craniopharyngiomas: a clinical and pathological review. *Cancer* 1976;37:1944–1952.

Submitted by: Andrew Mancall, M.D., and C. Roger Bird, M.D., Barrow Neurological Institute, Phoenix, Arizona; Rosalind B. Dietrich, M.B., Ch.B., Senior Editor.

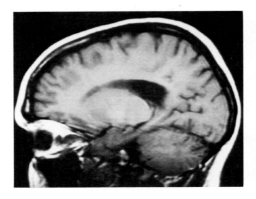
FIG. 26A. SE 700/11.

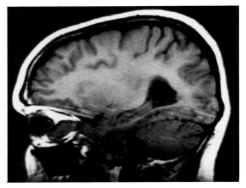
FIG. 26B. SE 700/11.

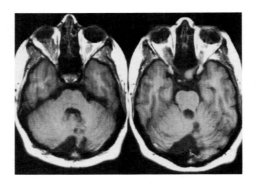
FIG. 26C. SE 450/15.

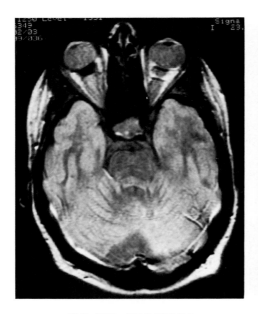
FIG. 26D. SE 2,500/30.

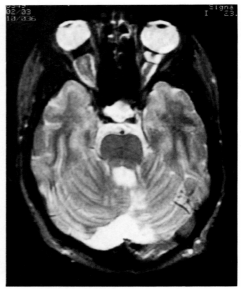
FIG. 26E. SE 2,500/90.

Clinical History

A 13-year-old female status post-resection of a posterior fossa meningioma with decreased visual acuity.

Findings

There is gross enlargement of both optic nerves, primarily involving the intraorbital portion of the right optic nerve and the extraorbital portion of the left optic nerve with extension to involve the left side of the optic chiasm. There may be slight enhancement of the enlarged right optic nerve.

Diagnosis

Bilateral optic nerve gliomas.

Discussion

Optic nerve gliomas are generally considered low-grade astrocytomas, although some authors believe they might actually represent hamartomatous lesions (1). Such tumors are found primarily in the young, with 60%–75% presenting by age 10 and 80%–90% by age 20 (1,2). Symptoms at presentation include optic atrophy, exophthalmos, and impaired extraocular eye muscle movements, with proptosis usually preceding loss of visual acuity (2). Tumor may spread posteriorly to involve the chiasm, optic tracts, and lateral geniculate bodies.

Optic nerve glioma represents an integral part of the neurofibromatosis 1 syndrome and has been well described by others (3,4).

MR demonstrates enlargement of the optic nerve with or without extension to involve the chiasm and optic tracts. Lesions are typically hypo- to isointense on T1-weighted images and iso- to hyperintense on T2-weighted images (2). Enhancement is variable and has been reported in as many as 50% of cases on CT, although the degree of enhancement is usually less intense than that expected with meningioma (5).

References

1. Alvord EC, Lofton S. Gliomas of the optic nerve or chiasm: outcome by patient's age, tumor site and treatment. *JNS* 1988;68:85–98.
2. Stark DD, Bradley WG. *Magnetic resonance imaging.* St. Louis: C. V. Mosby, 1988.
3. Aoki S, Barkovitch AJ, Nishimura K. Neurofibromatosis types 1 and 2: cranial MR findings. *Radiology* 1989;172:527–534.
4. National Institute of Health Consensus Development. Neurofibromatosis. *Arch Neurol* 1988;45:575–578.
5. Newton T, Hasso A, Dillon W. *Modern neuroradiology: computed tomography of the head and neck, vol. 3.* New York: Raven Press, 1988.

Submitted by: Andrew Mancall, M.D., and C. Roger Bird, M.D., Barrow Neurological Institute, Phoenix, Arizona; Rosalind B. Dietrich, M.B., Ch.B., Senior Editor.

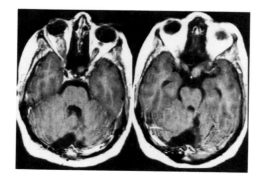

FIG. 26F. SE 450/15 with Gd-DTPA.

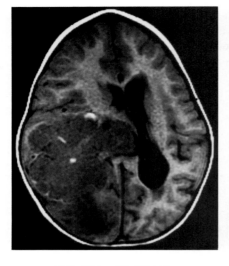

FIG. 27A. SE 750/16.

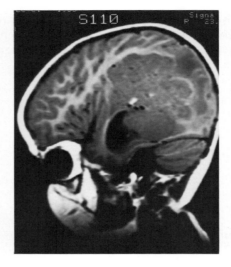

FIG. 27B. SE 700/16.

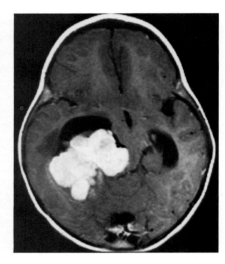

FIG. 27C. SE 2,500/30.

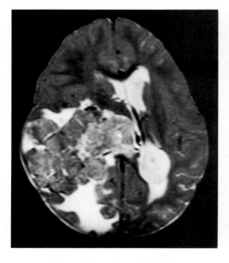

FIG. 27D. SE 2,500/90.

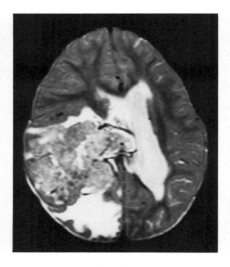

FIG. 27E. SE 2,500/90.

FIG. 27F. SE 750/16 with Gd-DTPA.

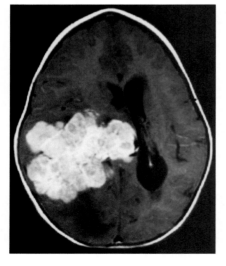

FIG. 27G. SE 750/16 with Gd-DTPA.

Clinical History

A 2-year-old female with vomiting, seizures, and ataxia.

Findings

There is a large, lobulated mass with its epicenter in the region of the atrium of the right lateral ventricle extending into the adjacent right parietal and posterior temporal regions. The mass demonstrates inhomogeneous signal intensity on both T1-W and T2-W images. A large amount of surrounding vasogenic edema is present with mass effect and midline shift to the left. There is intense and heterogeneous enhancement of the mass after gadolinium administration.

Diagnosis

Choroid plexus carcinoma.

Discussion

Choroid plexus carcinoma is a distinctly uncommon tumor comprising less than 0.5% of all intracranial primary tumors (1). The majority are found in patients in the first decade of life (most commonly between the ages of two and four years). Males are affected more frequently than females. Carcinomas are characterized by invasion of the adjacent parenchyma, and leptomeningeal dissemination is a notable feature (exceptional in benign choroid plexus papillomas) (2). Ventricular enlargement may be due to overproduction of CSF or blockage of CSF pathways by tumor spread. Malignant choroid plexus papilloma may be difficult to distinguish from medulloepithelioma or teratoma.

In general, the tumors are of intermediate signal intensity on T1-weighted images and may be of intermediate or increased signal intensity on T2-weighted images (3,4). There is usually intense enhancement following gadolinium-DTPA administration.

Differential considerations include benign choroid plexus papilloma and papillary ependymoma. The invasive nature of the choroid plexus carcinomas as well as its propensity to metastasize throughout the CSF space are clues to the correct diagnosis (4).

References

1. Russell DS, Rubenstein LJ. *Pathologic tumors of the nervous system,* 5th ed. Baltimore: Williams and Wilkins, 1989;401–403.
2. Okazaki H. *Fundamentals of neuropathology.* New York, Tokyo: Igaku-Shoin, 1983;200–203.
3. Stark D, Bradley W. *Magnetic resonance imaging.* St. Louis: C. V. Mosby, 1988;397.
4. Coates TL, Hinshaw DB, Peckman N. Pediatric choroid plexus neoplasms: MR, CT, and pathologic correlation. *Radiology* 1989;173:81.

Submitted by: Eric C. Flint, M.D., and C. Roger Bird, M.D., Barrow Neurological Institute, Phoenix, Arizona; Rosalind B. Dietrich, M.B., Ch.B., Senior Editor.

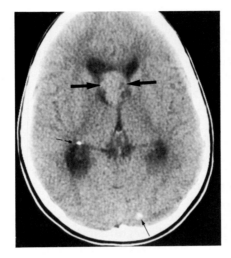

FIG. 28A. CT.

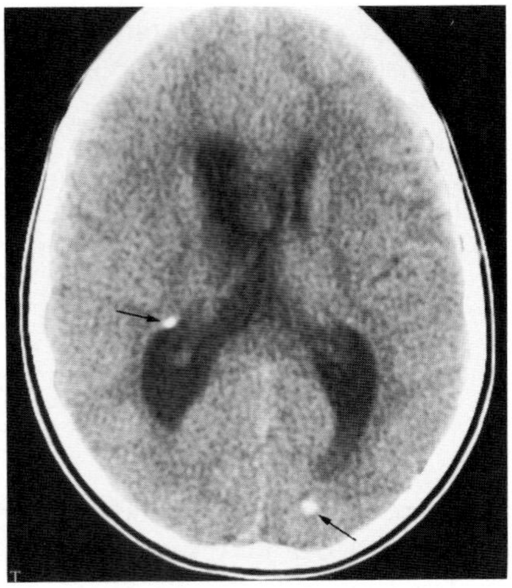

FIG. 28B. CT.

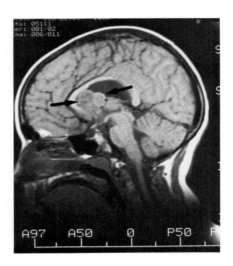

FIG. 28C. SE 600/20.

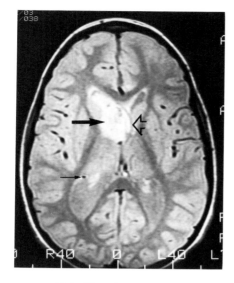

FIG. 28D. SE 2,727/20.

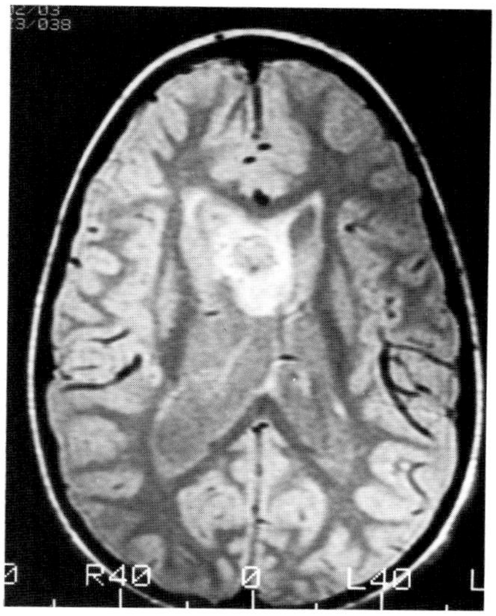

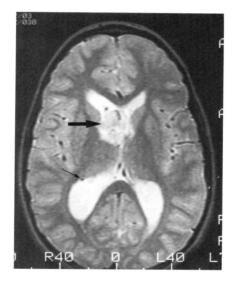

FIG. 28E. SE 2,727/20.

FIG. 28F. SE 2,727/70.

Clinical History

A 12-year-old, previously healthy girl presented with severe headache. On physical examination she was found to have papilledema.

Findings

CT scan shows hydrocephalus, intracranial calcifications (Figs. 28A and B, *small black arrows*), and an intraventricular mass, in the region of the foramen of Monro (Figs. 28A and B).

MRI scan was performed using T1-weighted sagittal and coronal image sequences and dual echo axial and coronal images. The sagittal midline image (Fig. 28C) delineates the mass in the anterior aspect of the ventricular system, extending anteriorly in the midline to the corpus callosum. The aqueduct is delineated and the fourth ventricle is normal in size and shape.

The axial and coronal images confirm that the mass (*large black arrows*) is in the right lateral ventricle (Figs. 28D, F, H and I). The septum pellucidum and adjacent interhemispheric vessels (Figs. 28D, H, and I, *open black arrows*) are displaced to the left of the midline.

On the T1-weighted sagittal and coronal images the mass has intermediate signal intensity and is clearly outlined by the low signal intensity of the CSF surrounding it on its superior aspect. The mass shows inhomogeneous signal on the axial scans. On the T2-weighted images, the mass has intermediate signal intensity and is outlined by high signal intensity CSF (Figs. 28F and G).

On MRI, the calcifications, which are subependymal in location, are markedly hypointense (Figs. 28D, F, *small black arrows*). They are less striking than the appearance of the calcifications on the CT scan.

Diagnosis

Tuberous sclerosis, with a giant cell astrocytoma arising in the region of the foramen of Monro.

Discussion

Tuberous sclerosis is a hereditary disease, first described by von Recklinghausen and later by Bourneville in more detail in 1880 (1). The disease is inherited as an autosomal dominant in approximately 20%–50% of cases, but sporadic cases are common. It is one of the phakomatoses, but is seen less frequently than neurofibromatosis. The clinical triad classically consists of adenoma sebaceum, seizures, and mental retardation. Seizures occur in 80%–90% of patients and mental retardation in approximately 60%.

Tuberous sclerosis is a dyshistogenesis in which there is an overgrowth of astrocytes (2). Hamartomas can involve all organs. Subungual fibromas, rhabdomyomas and sarcomas of the heart, and angiomyolipomas of the kidney may be present. Intracranially, the most common site is the cerebrum, but hamartomas may also be cortical. Hamartomas may also be present in the cerebellum, medulla, and spinal cord (1).

The four types of intracerebral lesions are cortical tubers, white matter abnormalities, subependymal nodules, and subependymal giant cell astrocytomas.

The cortical tubers are more commonly frontal than occipital and rare in the cerebellum. The lesions are located in the gyri, extending variably into white matter. They consist of giant cells with decreased myelin sheaths, and there is dense fibrillary gliosis. The tubers,

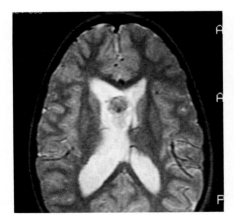

FIG. 28G. SE 2,727/70.

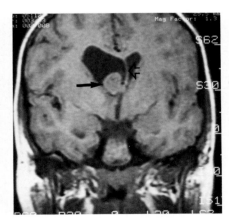

FIG. 28H. SE 667/20.

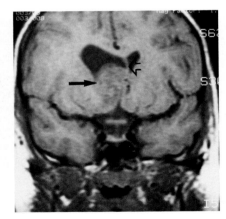

FIG. 28I. SE 667/20.

when present, are seen on MRI to have focal hypointensity to brain parenchyma on short TR sequence and are hyperintense on long TR, most likely due to the gliosis.

The white matter lesions also consist of clusters of heterotopic giant cells, orientated radially from the ventricular ependyma to the cortex, and show hyperintensity within the white matter on long TR sequences.

The subependymal nodules occur most commonly on the surface of the caudate nucleus and are also seen in the third and fourth ventricles. They project into the ventricles and also contain giant cells, but in this location are more often of the giant astrocyte type, and depositions of calcium are nearly always present. The calcification is better seen on CT than MR, but the location and contour of the nodules is typical of TS. They are isointense to white matter on short TR sequences and markedly hypointense to white matter with long TR spin-echo and gradient-echo sequences.

Malignant change of the hamartomas of the cerebrum is most common in the subependymal nodules closest to the foramen of Monro (1). The neoplasms are slow growing and histologically classified as giant cell astrocytomas. Subependymal and interventricular giant cell astrocytoma occurs in as many as 10% of cases with tuberous sclerosis (3). Obstructive hydrocephalus may occur, as in this case, secondary to location and/or change in size.

References

1. Rao KCVG, Harwood-Nash DC. In: Lee SH, Rao KCVG, eds. *Cranial computed tomography and MRI,* 2nd ed. New York: McGraw-Hill Inc., 1983, pp. 165–231.
2. Naidich TP, Zimmerman RA. In: Brant-Zawadski M, Norman D, eds. *Magnetic resonance imaging of the central nervous system.*
3. Braffman BH, Bilaniuk LT, Zimmerman RA. The central nervous system manifestations of the phakomatoses on MR. *Radiol Clin North Am* 1988;26.

Submitted by: Patricia E. Perry, M.D., Good Samaritan Regional Medical Center and Phoenix Children's Hospital, Phoenix, Arizona; Rosalind B. Dietrich, M.B., Ch.B., Senior Editor.

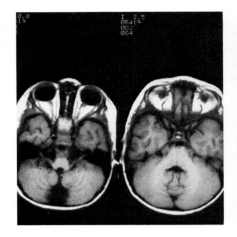

FIG. 29A. SE 450/15.

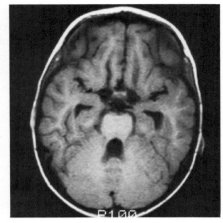

FIG. 29B. SE 450/15.

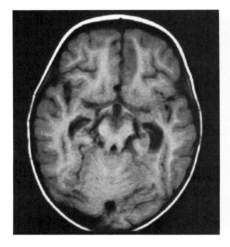

FIG. 29C. SE 450/15.

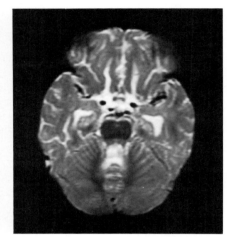

FIG. 29D. SE 2,500/90.

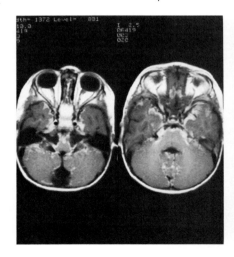

FIG. 29E. SE 450/15 with Gd-DTPA.

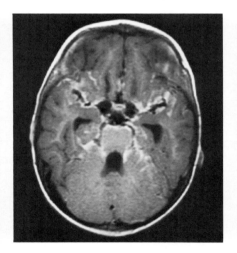

FIG. 29F. SE 450/15 with Gd-DTPA.

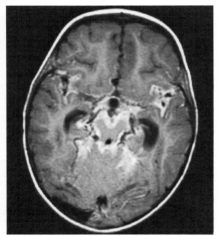

FIG. 29G. SE 450/15 with Gd-DTPA.

Clinical History

A 17-month-old female had a seizure following a course of chemotherapy for a rhabdomyosarcoma diagnosed at 7 months of age.

68

Findings

Moderate ventricular enlargement is noted, best seen on the axial T1-weighted images. After administration of gadolinium-DTPA, enhancement can be seen in the sylvian fissures and basilar cisterns and along the ventral aspect of the brain stem. No intraaxial lesion or abnormal enhancement is present.

Diagnosis

Carcinomatous meningitis.

Discussion

Carcinomatous meningitis or leptomeningeal spread of tumor is a diffuse infiltration of the meninges in a sheet-like fashion. Although the entire surface of the brain and cord may be involved, pathologically the ventral brain stem and suprasellar cisterns show the highest concentration of tumor (1). The meninges are thickened by a combination of tumor and often an associated inflammatory response. These meningeal changes are often inapparent on unenhanced MR images (2). Enhanced MR images are more sensitive than CT in demonstrating such findings (3). The differential diagnosis should include granulomatous or infectious meningitis.

Patients may present with symptoms of carcinomatous meningitis as the first sign of their malignancy (4).

On examination, the patient usually has signs and symptoms of disease at more than one site in the CNS and neurologic signs show more dysfunction than symptoms (1). The CSF evaluation is the most helpful test. The protein is usually elevated, the glucose low, but multiple samples may be necessary to demonstrate abnormal cytology. The mechanism of spread to the meninges appears to be a combination of (a) direct extension, (b) hematogenous seeding of the choroid, and (c) via thin-walled veins in the leptomeninges (4). Cranial nerve and spinal root symptoms are common (80%). The proposed pathogenesis of these symptoms is (a) demyelination and (b) ischemia due to occlusion of small perineural arteries (5).

References

1. Olsen ME, Chernik NL, Posner JB. Infiltration of the leptomeninges by systemic cancer. *Arch Neurol* 1974;30:122–137.
2. Davis PC, Friedman NC, Fry SM, Malko JA, Hoffman JC, Braun IF. Leptomeningeal metastasis: MR imaging. *Radiology* 1987;163:449–454.
3. Elster AD, DiPersio DA. Cranial postoperative site: assessment with contrast-enhanced MR imaging. *Radiology* 1990;174:93–98.
4. Little JR, Dale AJ, Okazaki H. Meningeal carcinomatosis. *Arch Neurol* 1974;30:138–143.
5. Case 14-1988. Case records of the Massachusetts General Hospital. *N Engl J Med* 1988;318:903–915.

Submitted by: Alex Mamourian, M.D., and C. Roger Bird, M.D., Barrow Neurological Institute, Phoenix, Arizona; Rosalind B. Dietrich, M.B., Ch.B., Senior Editor.

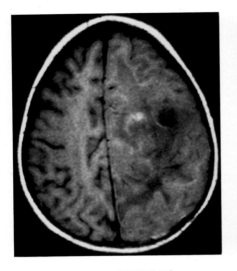 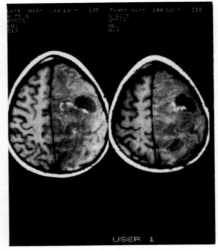 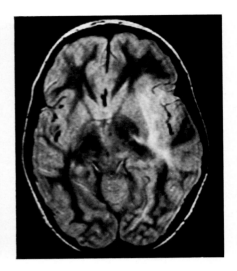

FIG. 30A. SE 750/16.   FIG. 30B. SE 750/16.   FIG. 30C. SE 2,500/30.

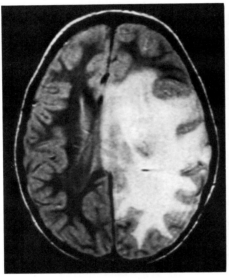
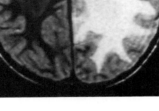

FIG. 30D. SE 2,500/30.   FIG. 30E. SE 2,500/90.

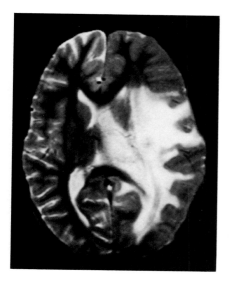

FIG. 30F. SE 2,500/90.

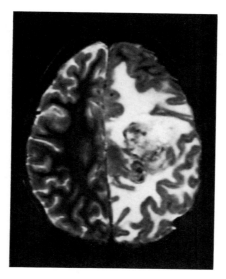

FIG. 30G. SE 2,500/90.

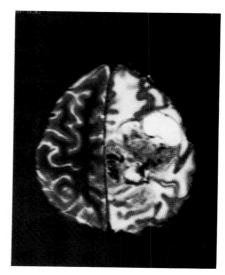

FIG. 30H. SE 2,500/90.

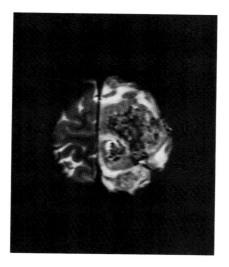

FIG 30I. SE 2,500/90.

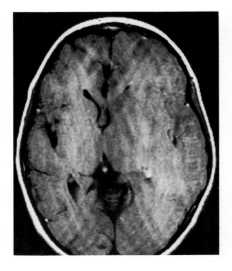 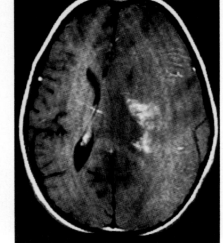 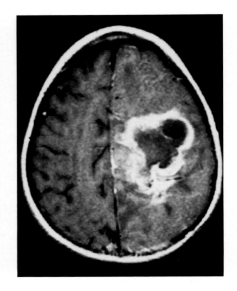

FIG. 30J. SE 733/16 with Gd-DTPA.　　FIG. 30K. SE 733/16 with Gd-DTPA.　　FIG. 30L. SE 733/16 with Gd-DTPA.

Clinical History

An 8-year-old female was diagnosed 2 years earlier with an anaplastic astrocytoma of the left parietal lobe. She was treated by subtotal surgical resection and focal radiation therapy.

Findings

There is a large inhomogeneous mass in the left parietal lobe. The mass demonstrates areas of necrosis, subacute hemorrhage, and extensive surrounding vasogenic edema. Following intravenous administration of gadolinium-DTPA, there is marked irregular enhancement of the mass.

Diagnosis

Radiation necrosis.

Discussion

Therapeutic radiation is commonly used to treat a wide variety of tumors of the CNS. Complications of this therapy commonly present as demyelination or necrosis (1,2). Demyelination typically presents within a few weeks or months following irradiation, whereas necrosis usually presents many months or even years following treatment (1,2).

Necrosis usually results after maximal doses of approximately 6,000 rads. Pathologically, necrosis develops due to endothelial proliferation and damage to the microvasculature (3). This is accompanied by breakdown of the blood-brain barrier (BBB) and perivascular inflammation.

On MRI radiation necrosis appears as a necrotic "mass" with surrounding edema. Hemorrhage and calcification may also be present. Since the BBB is disrupted there is usually abnormal enhancement following administration of gadolinium-DTPA. Such findings closely resemble residual or recurrent tumor; it is often difficult or impossible to distinguish radiation necrosis from tumor by MRI (1). Biopsy is usually necessary. Positron emission tomography may be helpful in this differentiation in that radiation necrosis is hypometabolic, and residual or recurrent tumor is usually hypermetabolic (4).

References

1. Dooms GC, Hecht S, Brant-Zawadzki M, Berthiamue Y, Norman D, Newton TH. Brain radiation lesions: MR imaging. *Radiology* 1986;158:149–155.
2. Tsuruda JS, Kortman KE, Bradley WG, Wheeler DC, Van Dalsem W, Bradley TP. Radiation effects on cerebral white matter: MR evaluation. *AJNR* 1987;8:431–437.
3. Okazaki H. *Fundamentals of neuropathology.* New York, Tokyo: Igaku-Shoin, 1983.
4. DiChiro G, Oldfield E, Wright DC, et al. Cerebral necrosis after radiotherapy and/or intraarterial chemotherapy for brain tumors: PET and neuropathologic studies. *AJNR* 1987;8:1083–1091.

Submitted by: C. Roger Bird, M.D., Barrow Neurological Institute, Phoenix, Arizona; Rosalind B. Dietrich, M.B., Ch.B., Senior Editor.

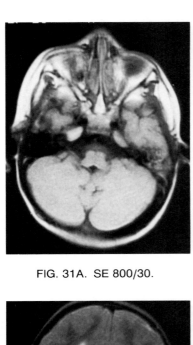

FIG. 31A. SE 800/30.

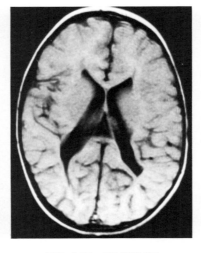

FIG. 31B. SE 800/30.

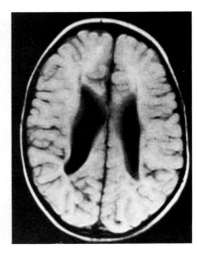

FIG. 31C. SE 800/30.

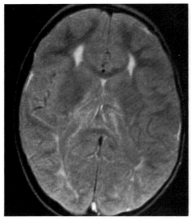

FIG. 31D. SE 2,000/85.

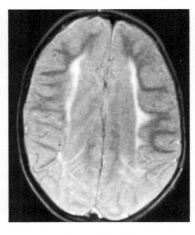

FIG. 31E. SE 2,000/85.

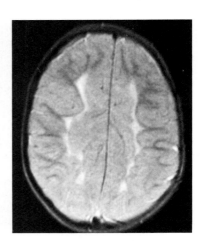

FIG. 31F. SE 2,000/85.

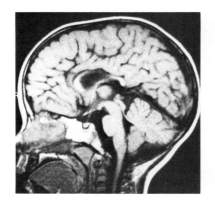

FIG. 31G. SE 500/30.

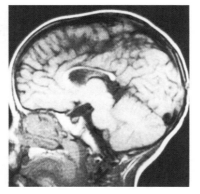

FIG. 31H. SE 500/30.

Clinical History

A 23-month-old boy, born prematurely, now being investigated for developmental delay.

74

Findings

On the T1-weighted images the lateral ventricles are mildly enlarged for a child of this age. Irregularity of the borders of the lateral ventricles is present, giving them a ragged contour. All parts of the corpus callosum are formed and on the sagittal T1-weighted sequence it demonstrates higher signal intensity than the adjacent cerebral parenchyma due to the deposition of myelin within it. The body of the corpus callosum, however, appears thinner than is normally seen in a child of this age.

On T2-weighted images areas of high signal intensity are identified in the periventricular white matter surrounding the lateral ventricles. Myelin deposition is delayed for a child of this age.

Diagnosis

Periventricular leukomalacia.

Discussion

Periventricular leukomalacia may develop in premature infants with cardiorespiratory disturbances and less commonly in term infants with congenital heart disease. In premature infants the watershed areas of the blood supply are in the periventricular regions. Therefore, in this group of infants, ischemic areas develop in the areas bordering the lateral ventricles, particularly in the white matter adjacent to the foramen of Monro or along the course of the optic radiations adjacent to the lateral aspect of the trigone. The lesions are frequently hemorrhagic, and regions of ischemic necrosis subsequently develop into areas of gliosis. In more severe cases, loss of brain substance occurs and discrete cystic areas can be identified within the periventricular white matter.

The MR findings of ragged ventricular borders and high signal intensity border in the adjacent white matter on T2-weighted images, as seen in this case, are characteristic of periventricular leukomalacia. In this entity, cystic white matter lesions demonstrating low signal intensity on T1-weighted images and high signal intensity on T2-weighted images may also be seen.

The thinning of the corpus callosum seen here is due to degeneration of transcallosal fibers occurring secondary to loss of adjacent white matter.

References

1. Wilson DA, Steiner RE. Periventricular leukomalacia; evaluation with MR imaging. *Radiology* 1986;160:507–511.
2. De Reuck J, Chatha AS, Richardson EP. Pathogenesis and evolution of periventricular leukomalacia in infancy. *Arch Neurol* 1972;27:229–236.
3. Flodmark O, Roland EH, Hill A, Whitfield MF. Periventricular leukomalacia: radiologic diagnosis. *Radiology* 1987;162:119–124.
4. Baker LL, Stevenson DK, Enzmann DR. Endstage periventricular leukomalacia: MR evaluation. *Radiology* 1988;168:809–815.

Submitted by: Rosalind B. Dietrich, M.B., Ch.B., Senior Editor.

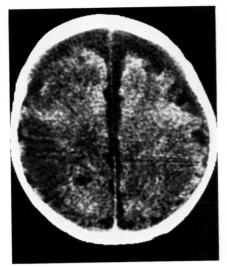

FIG. 32A. SE 800/28.

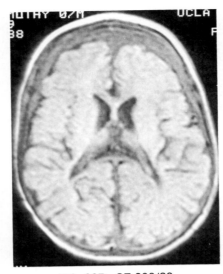

FIG. 32B. SE 800/28.

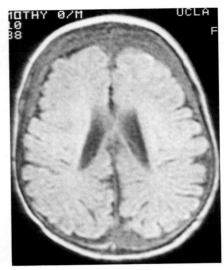

FIG. 32C. SE 800/28.

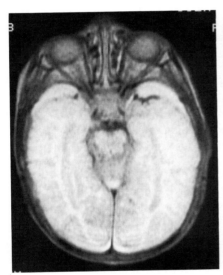

FIG. 32D. SE 2,000/84.

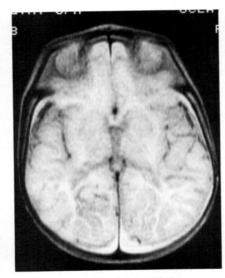

FIG. 32E. SE 2,000/84.

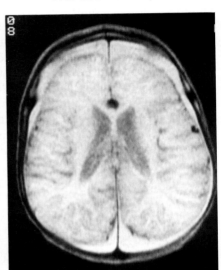

FIG. 32F. SE 2,000/84.

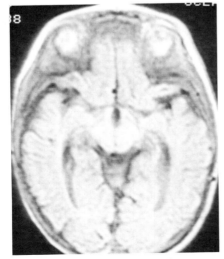

FIG. 32G. SE 800/28.

Clinical History

A 3-month-old boy with a sudden onset of seizures and blindness.

Findings

There are bilateral subdural fluid collections that demonstrate medium signal intensity on T1-weighted images and high signal intensity on T2-weighted images. On the T1-weighted images the fluid collections have higher signal intensity than the adjacent CSF. On T2-weighted images there is also a subtle loss of gray-white differentiation in the occipital lobes bilaterally.

CT scan performed the same day as the MR study demonstrates the same subdural fluid collections and also low density areas in the occipital lobes consistent with bilateral occipital infarction.

Diagnosis

Bilateral subdural hematomas and occipital infarctions secondary to child abuse.

Discussion

When subdural fluid collections are seen in young children, the differential diagnosis includes child abuse and benign hydrocephalus. Children with benign hydrocephalus usually present between the ages of 6 and 12 months with increasing head size and are developmentally normal for their age. In children with this diagnosis, the subdural collections are always bilaterally symmetric and have the same signal intensity as the adjacent CSF. By contrast, in children who have suffered child abuse, the fluid collections may be asymmetric in size and may demonstrate different signal intensity compared to each other and to the adjacent CSF. They may also be associated with other intracranial findings, some of which are extremely subtle, and also peripheral injuries.

The frequency of intracranial abnormalities in abused children is reported to range from 10%–44%, depending on the study. Evidence of several injuries of different ages anywhere in the body is needed to make the diagnosis. Intracranial findings seen include the presence of subdural hematomas, cortical contusions both hemorrhagic and nonhemorrhagic, shearing injuries, subarachnoid hemorrhages, and skull fractures. Diffuse axonal injury and subarachnoid hemorrhage may be caused by vigorous shaking, but cortical contusion and subdural hematomas with overlying bruising or skull fracture are more compatible with a direct blow.

Although both CT and MR can be used to evaluate children with child abuse, MR has been shown to be superior to CT in both detecting subdural hematomas and determining their ages. The presence on MR images of layers of subdural hemorrhage of differing ages or parenchymal hemorrhages of differing ages is extremely suggestive of nonaccidental injury.

Gradient-echo imaging is especially useful in demonstrating small areas of hemorrhage because of exquisite sensitivity to the presence of magnetic susceptibility effects of hemoglobin breakdown products and therefore may be particularly useful with battered children.

CT is better than MR at demonstrating overlying skull fractures or the presence of acute subarachnoid hemorrhage. It may more easily depict areas of nonhemorrhagic infarction in children under 8 months of age whose brains normally have a higher water content than older children. Because of this it may be extremely difficult to pick subtle increases in water content of the brain due to the presence of nonhemorrhagic infarction on T2-weighted images. Significant intracranial injuries, as demonstrated by MR or CT, in combination with a disproportionate history should be considered child abuse until proven otherwise.

References

1. Zimmerman RA, Bilaniuk LT, Bruce D, Schut L, Uzzell B, Goldberg HI. Computed tomography of craniocerebral injury in the abused child. *Radiology* 1979;130:687–690.
2. Sato YS, Yuh WTC, Smith WL, et al. Head injury in child abuse: evaluation with MR scanning. *Radiology* 1989;173:653–657.

Submitted by: Rosalind B. Dietrich, M.B., Ch.B., Senior Editor.

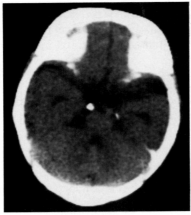

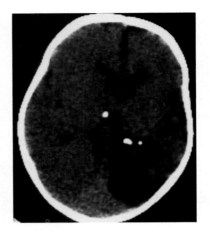

FIG. 33A. CT.

FIG. 33B. CT.

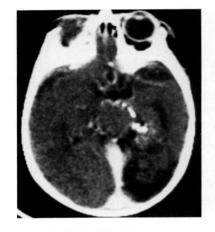
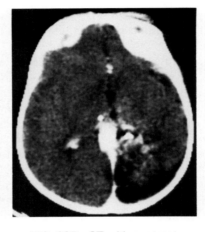
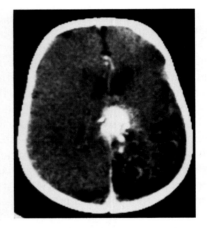

FIG. 33C. CT with contrast.

FIG. 33D. CT with contrast.

FIG. 33E. CT with contrast.

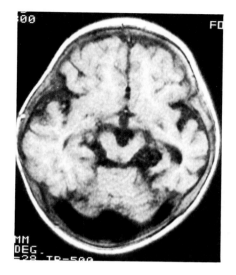

FIG. 33F. SE 500/28.

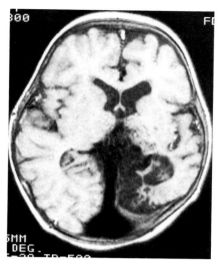

FIG. 33G. SE 500/28.

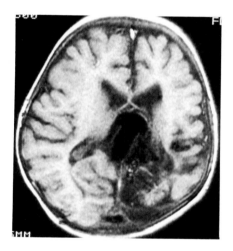

FIG. 33H. SE 300/28.

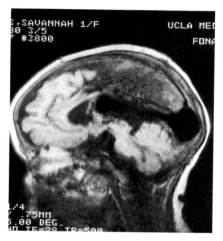

FIG. 33I. SE 500/28.

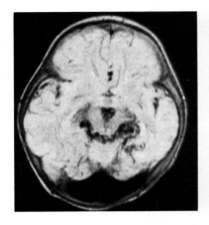 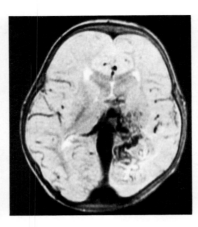 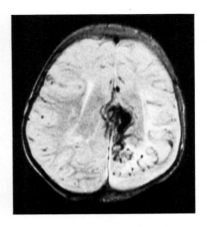

FIG. 33J. SE 2,000/84.   FIG. 33K. SE 2,000/84.   FIG. 33L. SE 2,000/84.

Clinical History

A 1-year-old girl who presented at birth with signs and symptoms of congestive heart failure. An echocardiogram was obtained that demonstrated no evidence of congenital heart disease.

Findings

CT scan (with and without contrast) performed at 2 months of age shows an extensive area of low density in the left parieto-occipital region. Discrete areas of calcification are seen bilaterally. Following administration of contrast, there are serpiginous areas of enhancement within the previously noted low density area and marked enhancement of a massively enlarged vein of Galen and straight sinus.

An MR study was obtained at 1 year of age. T1-weighted MR images demonstrate a large region of low signal intensity in the left parieto-occipital region. Within this region are serpiginous tubular structures consistent with blood vessels. On T2-weighted images the blood vessels show varied signal intensity. In some vessels high signal intensity is seen adjacent to the vessel wall. The dilated vein of Galen and straight sinus are again seen and are of low signal intensity.

Diagnosis

Vein of Galen malformation.

Discussion

Vein of Galen anomalies are rare arteriovenous malformations that occur due to the intrauterine development of connections between intracranial vessels and the vein of Galen. The cause of the malformations is not clear, but it has been suggested that they occur following the development of straight sinus thrombosis and subsequent recanalization (1).

Children with this anomaly may present either in the newborn period or later in childhood. Newborn infants frequently present with congestive heart failure, and on examination a loud intracranial bruit can be heard. Older children may present with evidence of hydrocephalus, seizures, or hemorrhage.

In such patients MR is useful in demonstrating the vascular anatomy and any regions of hemorrhage. MR cannot only demonstrate the extent of the anomaly but can also demonstrate its vascular nature. It will also show any associated areas of infarction or hemorrhage. Depending on the velocity of blood through the malformation and the presence or absence of thrombosis, different signal intensities may be seen within the vessels of the malformation.

As the majority of the vessels usually contain fast-flowing blood, a signal void is usually present within them. The signal intensity of thrombus deposition within them will of course vary depending on its age. Acute thrombus will demonstrate low signal intensity on T2-weighted images, whereas subacute thrombus will have high signal intensity on T1-weighted images and low or high signal on T2-weighted images, depending on whether the red cells are still intact or have lysed.

References

1. Lasjaunias P, Ter Brugge K, Lopez-Ibor L, et al. The role of dural anomalies in vein of Galen aneurysms: report of six cases and review of the literature. *AJNR* 1987;8:185–192.
2. Hoffman HJ, Chuang S, Hendrick EB, Humphreys RP. Aneurysms of the vein of Galen. Experience at the Hospital for Sick Children, Toronto. *J Neurosurg* 1982;57:316–322.
3. Amacher AL, Shillito J Jr. The syndromes and surgical treatment of aneurysms of the great vein of Galen. *J Neurosurg* 1973;39:89–98.
4. Roosen N, Schirmer M, Lins E, et al. MRI of an aneurysm of the vein of Galen. *AJNR* 1986;7:733–735.
5. Rao KCVG, Lee SH. Cerebrovascular anomalies. In: Stark DD, Bradley WG, eds. *Magnetic resonance imaging.* St. Louis: C. V. Mosby, 1988;473–505.

Submitted by: Rosalind B. Dietrich, M.B., Ch.B., Senior Editor.

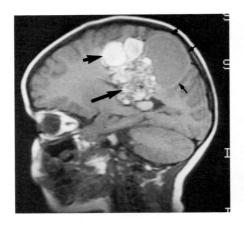

FIG. 34A. SE 600/20.

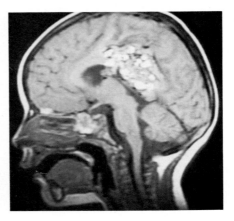

FIG. 34B. SE 600/20.

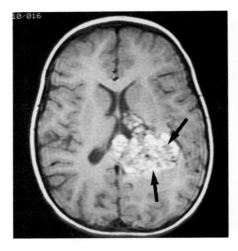

FIG. 34C. SE 600/20.

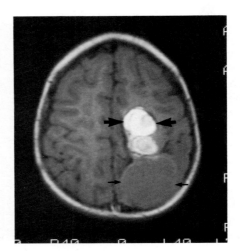

FIG. 34D. SE 600/20.

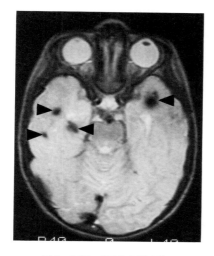

FIG. 34E. SE 2,500/70.

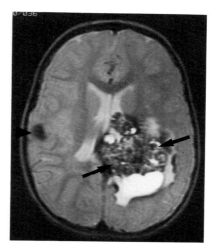

FIG. 34F. SE 2,500/70.

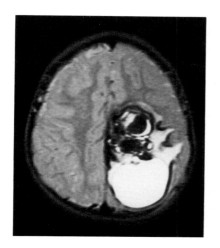

FIG. 34G. SE 2,500/70.

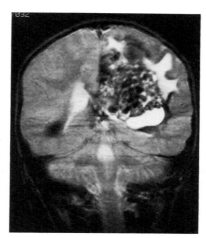

FIG. 34H. SE 2,500/80.

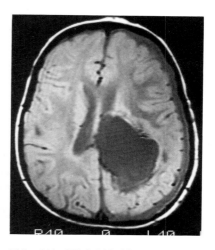

FIG. 34I. SE 2,500/20. Postoperative.

Clinical History

A 2-year-old Mexican-American girl, presented with twitching of the right hand, following a seizure.

Findings

MR images show a left parasagittal vascular mass involving the corpus callosum and adjacent cerebral hemisphere (Figs. 34A and D, *large black arrows*). On the short TR sequences there is a mixture of serpiginous areas (Figs. 34A, C, and F, *long black arrows*) of low signal consistent with flowing blood, scattered focal areas of hypointensity corresponding with calcification (seen on prior CT scan), large rounded areas of hyperintense signal consistent with stagnant blood with intact red blood cells (Figs. 34A and D, *short black arrows*), and central and peripheral low signal corresponding to deposition of hemosiderin.

There is a large rounded area of intermediate signal intensity on short TR, which shows high signal on long TR posterior to the vascular mass described (Figs. 34A and D, *small black arrows*), and this is consistent with a cyst containing proteinaceous material.

Multiple other areas of low signal intensity are scattered throughout the cerebrum (more obvious on the long TR sequences) consistent with previous hemorrhage (Figs. 34E and F, *black arrowheads*).

Note is made that for a lesion of this size, there is relatively little mass effect and no surrounding edema.

Angiography was performed following the MR showed sparse vascularity of the lesion.

Diagnosis

Cerebral cavernous hemangioma in a Mexican-American patient.

Discussion

Vascular malformations consist of four groups of developmental anomalies of the vascular system: capillary telangiectasis, cavernous hemangioma, arteriovenous malformations (AVMs), and venous malformation (1).

An intracranial malformation may have mass effect and there may be progressive destruction of adjacent brain tissue, but there is no proliferation of neural tissue, i.e., these abnormalities are not neoplasms (1).

Cavernous hemangiomas are the rarest form of vascular malformation, but intracranial cavernous hemangiomas (ICHs) are of clinical importance because they frequently present with seizures (1). The ICHs consist of clusters of sinusoids lined with endothelium, containing stagnant blood. There is no intervening neural tissue. Thrombosis, calcification, and hemorrhage can all occur. Lesions are multiple in as many as one-third of cases. ICHs are usually angiographically occult (3).

On MR, distinction between ICH, thrombosed AVMs, and capillary telangiectasis may not be possible, so the group of abnormalities may be referred to as occult cerebrovascular malformations (OCVM) or cryptic malformations (2).

On SE MR, OCVMs show the following appearances, which are virtually diagnostic and may make angiography unnecessary: (a) a heterogeneous, predominantly high signal corresponding to areas of hemorrhage, (b) a peripheral hypointense ring indicating deposition of hemosiderin, (c) no mass effect or edema, and (d) no demonstrable feeding arteries or draining veins (2).

Larger ICHs will of course, in the case described, have mass effect per se from size alone.

Differential diagnosis of ACVMs from hemorrhagic neoplasm may be difficult in the presence of acute hemorrhage. Serial MR scans would, however, show evolution of hematoma distinct from neoplasm.

Surgery in this patient demonstrated an AVM that was resected, and histology showed large thin-walled channels in a predominantly cavernous hemangioma. A post-operative study (Fig. 34I) shows a porencephalic cyst at the site of the resection.

A familial incidence of cerebral cavernous malformations has been described and is transmitted in an autosomal dominant fashion, with an increased frequency among Mexican-American families. In these patients it also has a high incidence of multiple lesions. This is important because the lesion may present with seizures and is well delineated on MRI. MRI is also the study of choice for screening relatives of patients with known disease.

References

1. Terbrugge K, Rao KCVG, Lee H. Cerebral vascular anomalies. In: Lee SH, Rao KCVG, eds. *Cranial computed tomography and MRI,* 2nd ed. New York: McGraw-Hill, 1983, pp. 607–643.
2. Atlas W. Intracranial vascular malformations and aneurysms: current imaging applications. *Radiol Clin North Am* 1988;26:821–826.
3. Cohen HCM, Tucker WS, Humphreys RP, et al. Angiographically cryptic histologically verified cerebro-vascular malformations. *Neurosurgery* 1982;10:837.
4. Rigamonti D, Hadley MN, Drayer BP, et al. Cerebral cavenous malformations: Incidence and familial occurrence. *N Engl J Med* 1988;319:343–347.

Submitted by: Patricia E. Perry, M.D., Good Samaritan Regional Medical Center and Phoenix Children's Hospital, Phoenix, Arizona; Rosalind B. Dietrich, M.B., Ch.B., Senior Editor.

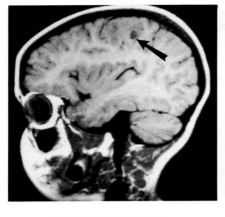

FIG. 35A. SE 617/20.

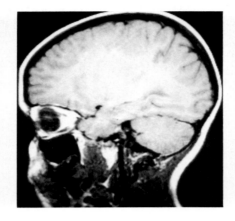

FIG. 35B. SE 617/20.

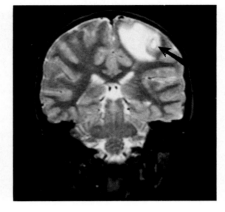

FIG. 35C. SE 3,273/80.

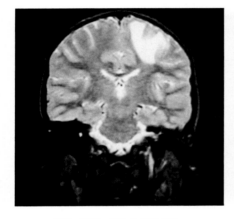

FIG. 35D. SE 3,273/80.

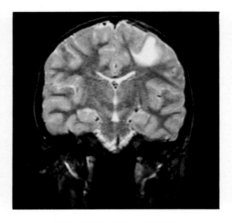

FIG. 35E. SE 3,273/80.

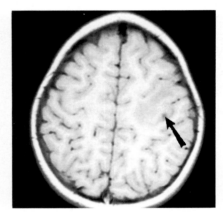

FIG. 35F. SE 600/20.

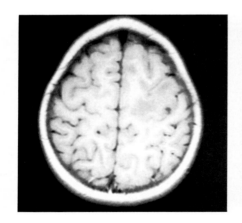

FIG. 35G. SE 600/20.

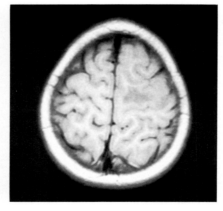

FIG. 35H. SE 600/20.

Clinical History

An 8-year-old girl with new onset seizures.

Findings

On the axial T2-weighted images there is an area of high signal intensity in the left parietal region. Within this area there is a small, round lesion with a high signal intensity center and a lower signal intensity rim (*arrow*). On axial and sagittal T1-weighted images the central lesion has low signal intensity and the surrounding area has medium signal intensity. These findings are consistent with a cystic lesion with surrounding edema. On the sagittal T1-weighted images the small cystic lesion has a high signal intensity dot within it.

Diagnosis

Parenchymal cysticercosis.

Discussion

The single area of high signal intensity seen on T2-weighted images is a nonspecific finding and may be due to the presence of a tumor, an infectious process, or infarction. The identification of the small cystic lesion within it, however, clinches the diagnosis of cysticercosis.

Neurocysticercosis is due to infestation by the larvae of the tapeworm *Taenia solium* and is usually acquired by the accidental ingestion of tapeworm eggs from fecal-contaminated substances.

The parenchymal type is the most common, accounting for 80% of cases. Other types described are intraventricular, racemose, and leptomeningeal. Infected patients may present with seizures, hydrocephalus (due to obstruction by intraventricular or basal cistern cysts or by leptomeningeal involvement), or infarction secondary to vasculitis.

On MR images active parenchymal lesions are usually located in the gray matter. The lesions demonstrate a high signal intensity center with a lower signal intensity surrounding rim on T2-weighted images and often have a surrounding area of edema. On T1-weighted images a high signal intensity scolex may be seen within the low signal intensity cyst and active lesions show rim enhancement following gadolinium-DTPA administration. Once the larvae die, the lesions become calcified and therefore demonstrate low signal intensity on MR images and no longer enhance.

References

1. Suss RA, Maravilla KR, Thompson J. MR imaging of intracranial cysticercosis: comparison with CT and anatomopathologic features. *AJNR* 1986;7:235–242.
2. Martinez HR, Rangel-Guerra R, Elizondo G. MR imaging in neurocysticercosis: a study of 56 cases. *AJNR* 1989; 10:1011–1015.

Submitted by: Rosalind B. Dietrich, M.B., Ch.B., Senior Editor.

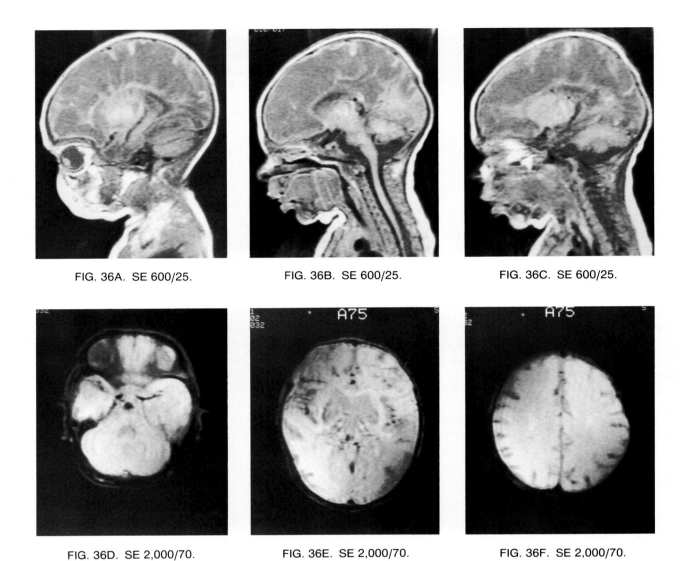

FIG. 36A. SE 600/25.

FIG. 36B. SE 600/25.

FIG. 36C. SE 600/25.

FIG. 36D. SE 2,000/70.

FIG. 36E. SE 2,000/70.

FIG. 36F. SE 2,000/70.

Clinical History

A 1-month-old boy with fever, lethargy, and seizures.

Findings

T1-weighted sagittal images demonstrate diffuse low signal intensity throughout the cerebral hemispheres; the signal intensity of the cerebellum and brain stem remains normal. On axial T2-weighted images the cerebral hemispheres demonstrate diffuse high signal intensity with total loss of the gray-white matter differentiation.

Diagnosis

Congenital herpes simplex encephalitis.

Discussion

Most cases of congenital herpes result from exposure of the child to herpetic genital lesions as it passes through the birth canal. Symptoms develop within the first month of life and may be neurologic (seizures, lethargy, and fever) or visceral (cyanosis, jaundice, fever, and respiratory distress). The disease may be fatal and surviving children have a poor prognosis.

The MR findings are consistent with the presence of diffuse cerebral edema. The widespread involvement of both the gray and white matter, together with the clinical history, favors an infectious process as the underlying etiology, most likely a virus. Although diffuse anoxia, in its acute stage, may also have the same MR findings, such a diagnosis is less likely in this child, who had a normal birth history and is febrile.

Initially, MR images of children with herpes encephalitis demonstrate patchy areas of low signal intensity on T1-weighted and high signal intensity on T2-weighted sequences, becoming more widespread with time. Meningeal enhancement may be seen following gadolinium-DTPA administration. Later the development of diffuse cerebral atrophy, with areas of porencephaly and gliosis, may be seen.

Reference

1. Noorbehesht B, Enzmann DR, Sullinder W, Bradley JS, Arvin AM. Neonatal herpes simplex encephalitis: correlation of clinical and CT findings. *Radiology* 1987;162:813–819.

Submitted by: Rosalind B. Dietrich, M.B., Ch.B., Senior Editor.

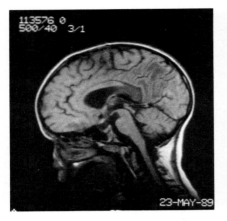

FIG. 37A. SE 2,500/80.

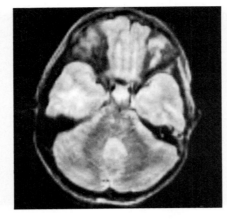

FIG. 37B. SE 2,500/80.

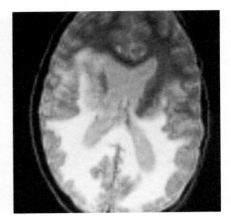

FIG. 37C. SE 2,500/80.

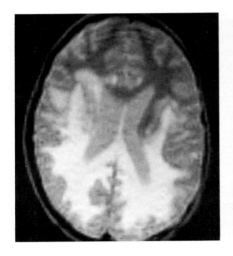

FIG. 37D. SE 2,500/80.

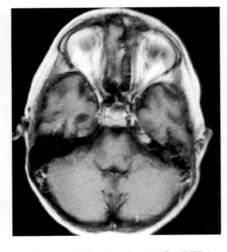

FIG. 37E. SE 500/30 with Gd-DTPA.

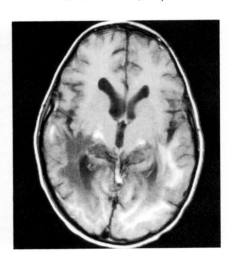

FIG. 37F. SE 500/30 with Gd-DTPA.

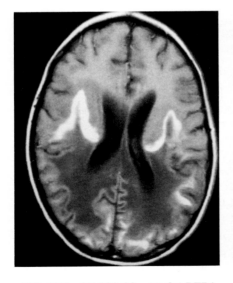

FIG. 37G. SE 500/30 with Gd-DTPA.

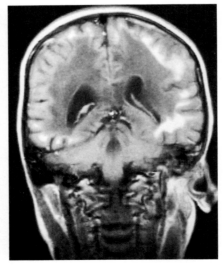

FIG. 37H. SE 500/30 with Gd-DTPA.

Clinical History

An 8-year-old boy with decreasing vision, clumsiness, and behavioral difficulties.

Findings

MR images obtained prior to administration of gadolinium-DTPA demonstrate large, confluent areas of abnormal signal intensity in the parieto-occipital white matter. These areas demonstrate high signal intensity on T2-weighted images and low signal intensity on T1-weighted images. T1-weighted images obtained following administration of gadolinium-DTPA show areas of enhancement only along the periphery of the areas of abnormal signal intensity. Involvement of the splenium and posterior body of the corpus callosum is also seen, and the lateral ventricles are mildly dilated.

Diagnosis

Adrenoleukodystrophy (ALD).

Discussion

These findings together with the clinical history are consistent with a leukodystrophy. Leukodystrophies are metabolic diseases due to inborn errors of metabolism. In this group of diseases, the abnormal accumulation of catabolites within the white matter of the brain results in irreversible damage to the myelin present within the white matter leading to a progressive and devastating clinical course. Although it is often difficult or impossible to differentiate the different leukodystrophies based on their MR findings, a relatively specific pattern of involvement occurs in several of the diseases. In this particular case it can be seen that the pattern of white matter involvement has started dorsally and is progressing ventrally. Also, there is peripheral enhancement of the involved areas. These findings are relatively specific for the entity of ALD.

ALD is a lipidosis, and the serum of affected children demonstrates a high percentage of fatty acids with long chains. Their myelin also shows marked elevation of cholesterol esters with very long chain fatty acids. There are several variants of ALD. The most common is an X-linked disorder involving both the adrenal cortex and the white matter of the CNS. Symptoms such as gradual gait disturbance or mild intellectual impairment usually develop between 5 and 9 years of age in affected boys. Progression of the disease is usually rapid with the development of seizures, hypotonia, visual complaints, and difficulty in swallowing. Symptoms of adrenal insufficiency may precede or follow the neurologic ones. Neonatal ALD is autosomal recessive and affected children demonstrate severe developmental delay and failure to thrive from birth onward. Neurologic symptoms are seen in conjunction with hepatomegaly and sometimes jaundice. In neonatal ALD there are no clinical signs of adrenal insufficiency. The entity of adrenomyeloneuropathy is thought to be an adult variant of ALD.

References

1. Kumar AJ, Rosenbaum AE, Naidu S, et al. Adrenoleukodystrophy: correlating MR imaging with CT. *Radiology* 1987;165:497–504.
2. Moser HW, Moser ARE, Singh I, O'Neill BP. Adrenoleukodystrophy: survey of 303 cases: biochemistry, diagnosis and therapy. *Ann Neurol* 1984;16:628–641.

Submitted by: Rosalind B. Dietrich, M.B., Ch.B., Senior Editor.

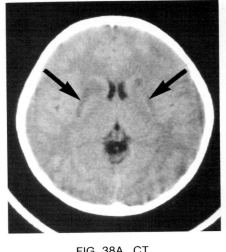

FIG. 38A. CT.

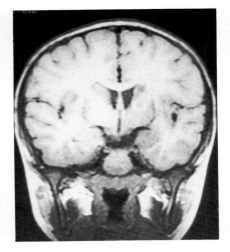

FIG. 38B. SE 617/20.

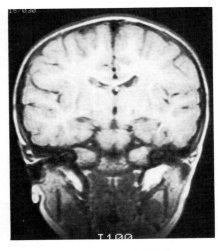

FIG. 38C. SE 617/20.

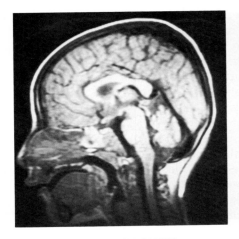

FIG. 38D. SE 617/20.

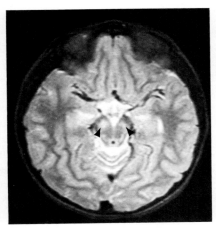

FIG. 38E. SE 3,000/80.

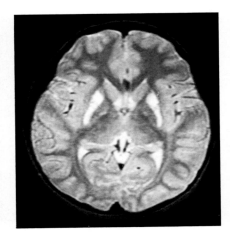

FIG. 38F. SE 3,000/80.

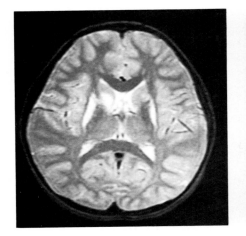

FIG. 38G. SE 3,000/80.

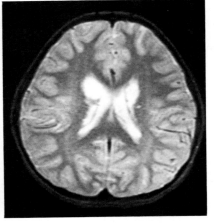

FIG. 38H. SE 3,000/80.

Clinical History

A 6-year-old girl with blindness and inability to walk since 3 years of age.

Findings

CT scan demonstrates areas of low signal intensity in the putamina bilaterally (*arrows*). On the T2-weighted axial MR images these areas demonstrate high signal intensity. In addition, areas of high signal intensity are also seen in the red nuclei (*arrowheads*).

Diagnosis

Leigh's disease (subacute necrotizing encephalopathy).

Discussion

The differential diagnosis of bilateral high signal intensity areas in the basal ganglia includes Leigh's disease, Wilson's disease, mitochondrial encephalopathies, and anoxic-ischemic events secondary to total asphyxiation. Children with Wilson's disease usually present with hepatic symptoms and in addition to the basal ganglia involvement, they may also show thalamic involvement. The mitochondrial encephalomyopathies are multisystem diseases; diagnosis is confirmed following muscle biopsy. In children who have suffered total asphyxia, areas of high signal intensity are frequently seen in the putamina together with the globus pallidi and anterior thalami bilaterally.

Leigh's disease is an autosomal recessive disease that first presents in infancy or early childhood. Symptoms are frequently nonspecific and include hypotonia and seizures in infants, and ataxia, dysarthria, ophthalmoplegia, and nystagmus in older children. Affected children demonstrate a progressive downhill course resulting in death within a few years of presentation.

Classically, MR scans of affected children demonstrate areas of low signal intensity on T1-weighted images and high signal intensity on T2-weighted images in the regions of the caudate, putamen, periaqueductal gray matter, and less commonly, the cerebral white matter.

References

1. Geyer CA, Sartor KJ, Prendsky AJ, Abramson CL, Hodges FJ, Gado MH. Leigh's disease: CT and MR in five cases. *J Comput Assist Tomogr* 1988;12:40–44.
2. Davis PC, Hoffman JC, Braun IF et al. MR of Leigh's Disease (subacute necrotizing encephalomyelopathy). *AJNR* 1987;8:71–75.

Submitted by: Rosalind B. Dietrich, M.B., Ch.B., Senior Editor.

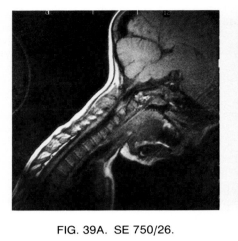

FIG. 39A. SE 750/26.

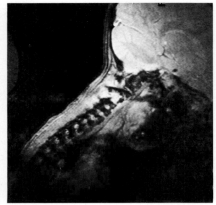

FIG. 39B. SE 517/18.

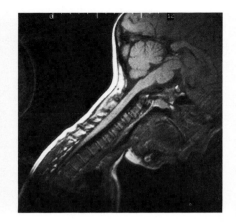

FIG. 39C. SE 750/26.

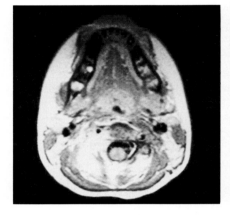

FIG. 39D. SE 683/26 with Gd-DTPA.

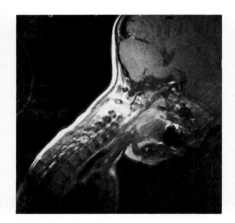

FIG. 39E. SE 750/26 with Gd-DTPA.

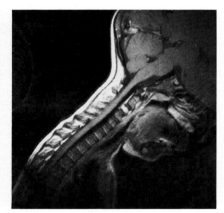

FIG. 39F. SE 750/26 with Gd-DTPA.

Clinical History

A 5-year-old white female with complains of pain and stiffness in the neck for several weeks.

Findings

There is a large area of abnormality that involves the body, right pedicle, and both laminae of the third cervical vertebra. There is a very large associated soft tissue mass that lies behind both sides of the vertebra and extends on the right side to the anterior margin of the vertebral body. T1-weighted pulse sequence (Fig. 39A) shows poorly defined swelling of soft tissues. T2-weighted gradient-echo image (Fig. 39B) shows increased signal intensity in the soft tissues and C3 vertebra. The spinal cord is normal (Fig. 39C). T1-weighted images after gadolinium administration (Figs. 39D–F) show a very large soft tissue abnormality with moderately uniform marked enhancement. There is also enhancement from the bony component of the lesion.

Diagnosis

Langerhans' cell histiocytosis (histiocytosis X).

Discussion

There are no specific features to suggest the correct diagnosis, but this diagnosis should always be considered with any lesion of the spine in children. Biopsy is needed to confirm the diagnosis. The MR findings of Langerhans' cell histiocytosis are nonspecific. High signal intensity on T2-weighted images or enhancement with gadolinium-DTPA administration is well recognized. The very extensive soft tissue abnormality and the lack of collapse of the vertebral body are unusual findings seen in this patient.

Differentiation of bone and soft tissue components of the lesion were much better demonstrated on CT.

Other considerations in the differential diagnosis would include malignant tumors such as osteogenic sarcoma and Ewing's sarcoma, but the patient is very young for these lesions as well as for lymphoma or rhabdomyosarcoma, both of which, however, should be considered. Osteomyelitis with extension into the soft tissues could have a very similar appearance and cannot be excluded.

Reference

1. Silverman FN. Histiocytosis. In: *Caffey's pediatric X-ray diagnosis.* Silverman F, Kuhn J, eds. Chicago: Year Book Publishers, 1985; pp. 325–327, 859.

Submitted by: Mervyn D. Cohen, M.B., Ch.B., Riley Hospital for Children, Indiana University Medical Center, Indianapolis, Indiana; Rosalind B. Dietrich, M.B., Ch.B., Senior Editor.

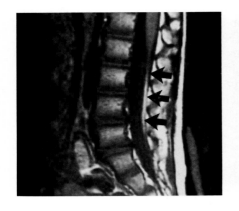

FIG. 40A. SE 550/20.

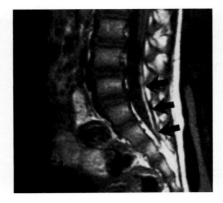

FIG. 40B. SE 550/20.

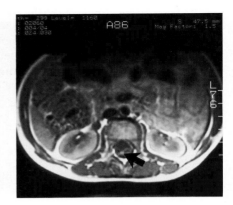

FIG. 40C. SE 750/20.

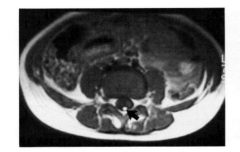

FIG. 40D. SE 750/20.

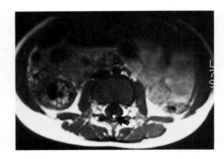

FIG. 40E. SE 750/20.

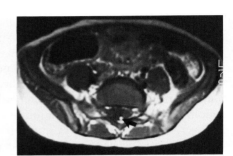

FIG. 40F. SE 750/20.

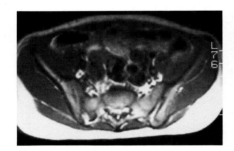

FIG. 40G. SE 750/20.

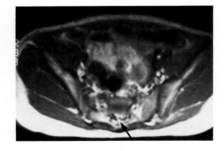

FIG. 40H. SE 750/20.

Clinical History

A 2-year-old girl presented with an unusual gait and urinary frequency.

Findings

On the sagittal T1-weighted images of the lumbosacral spine the filum terminale is thickened and has a signal intensity consistent with fatty infiltration (Figs. 40A and B, *arrows*). This is confirmed on the axial T1-weighted images (Figs. 40D–F, *arrow*), which show the filum to be 3–4 mm in diameter. The thickened fatty filum can be followed to its point of departure from the thecal sac in the midsacral region (Fig. 40H, *arrow*). The tip of the conus medullaris lies at the mid-L2 level (Fig. 40C, *arrow*).

Diagnosis

Fibrolipoma of the filum terminale.

Discussion

The caudal tip of the spinal cord ascends within the spinal canal due to the different growth rates of the spinal cord and the bony spine. In the newborn, the spinal cord may be as low as the body of L3. By 3 months of age, it should lie at about the L1–2 level. A low-lying cord is defined as one in which the tip of the conus medullaris lies below the L2 level: The cord is usually tethered by a thickened filum terminale that may be infiltrated by fat or an intraspinal mass such as a lipoma or dermoid tumor. A normal filum is uniform in thickness and less than 2 mm in diameter throughout its length. Proximally, the filum lies within the thecal sac. It then pierces the dura to insert on the dorsal surface of the first coccygeal vertebra. The thickening of the filum may be secondary to fibrotic tissue alone or to fatty infiltration (fibrolipoma). Thickening of the filum is usually associated with a low-lying cord, but occasionally it is not. Spina bifida occulta is frequently associated as is kyphoscoliosis in 25% of cases of thickened filum. Clinical findings include bladder dysfunction, club feet, back pain, sensory changes, and radiculopathy.

MRI with T1-weighted sequences is excellent for evaluating the filum and cord position. The thickened filum has signal intensity similar to nerve roots unless fatty infiltration is present to shorten T1. Axial images are best for determining the size of the filum as well as the precise location of the tip of the conus medullaris. Partial volume averaging may make it difficult to determine the exact size of the filum as well as the presence of fat on sagittal images. T2 imaging is usually not necessary.

References

1. Barkovich AJ, Naidich TP. Congenital anomalies of the spine. In: Barkovich AJ, ed. *Contemporary neuroimaging: pediatric neuroimaging,* vol. 1. New York: Raven Press, 1990;227–271.
2. Byrd SE. Radiologic evaluation of the pediatric spine. In: Poznanski AK, Kirkpatrick JA, eds. *Syllabus: a categorical course in diagnostic radiology, pediatric radiology.* Oak Brook, IL: RSNA, 1989;247–260.
3. De La Paz RL. Congenital anomalies of the spine and spinal cord. In: Enzmann DR, De La Paz RL, Rubin JB, eds. *Magnetic resonance of the spine.* St. Louis: C. V. Mosby, 1990;176–236.
4. Naidich TP, McLone DG. Congenital pathology of the spine and spinal cord. In: Taveras JM, Ferucci JT, eds. *Radiology: diagnosis-imaging-intervention,* vol. 3. Philadelphia: J. B. Lippincott, 1986, Ch. 103, pp. 1–23.

Submitted by: Robert A. Breit M.D., and Sharon E. Byrd M.D., Children's Memorial Hospital and Northwestern University Medical School, Chicago, Illinois; Rosalind B. Dietrich, M.B., Ch.B., Senior Editor.

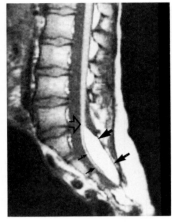
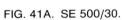
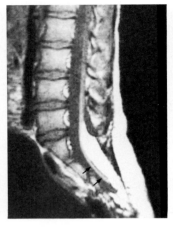
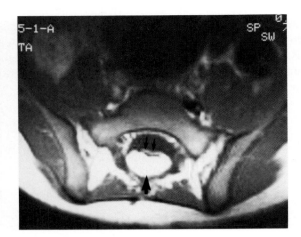

FIG. 41A. SE 500/30.   FIG. 41B. SE 500/30.   FIG. 41C. SE 600/30.

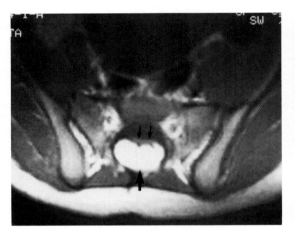
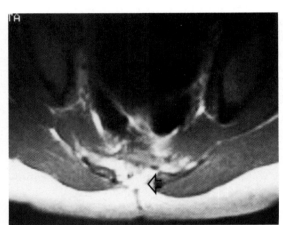

FIG. 41D. SE 600/30.   FIG. 41E. SE 600/30.

Clinical History

A 10-year-old boy had a lumbosacral dermal sinus tract resected at the age of 14 months.

Findings

Sagittal (SE 500/30) and axial (SE 600/30) images are presented. The spinal cord is tethered (Fig. 41A, *open arrow*) to a bright signal mass consistent with a lipoma (Figs. 41A and D, *arrow*) in the lumbosacral region. The mass lies dorsal to and is attached to the flattened continuation of the spinal cord, the neural placode (Figs. 41A–D, *small arrows*). The lipoma is contiguous with the subcutaneous fat through a lower sacral spina bifida defect (Fig. 41E, *open arrow*).

Diagnosis

Lipomyelomeningocele (LMM).

Discussion

There are three groups of spinal lipomas: intradural lipomas (4%), LMMs (84%), and fibrolipomas of the filum terminale (12%). The first two groups are thought to result from the premature separation of the neuroectoderm from the cutaneous ectoderm prior to neural tube closure. This allows the mesenchyme to approach the ependymal surface of the neural tube, preventing its closure, and resulting in open neural tissue, the "neural placode." The ependymal surface induces the mesenchyme to differentiate into fat dorsal to the cord, while normal meninges and bone still form from mesenchyme ventrally. Anatomically, LMMs are identical to myeloceles and myelomeningoceles except LMMs have the lipoma attached to the dorsal surface of the unclosed neural tissue and the overlying skin is intact. The lipoma is always contiguous with the subcutaneous fat through the spina bifida defect. Dura attaches to the lateral border of the placode at the junction of the lipoma and placode; thus, the dorsal surface of the nervous tissue abuts the lipoma and is extradural.

The lipoma can extend upward within the spinal canal to form an epidural lipoma or into the central canal of the spinal cord itself.

LMMs generally occur in the lumbosacral region and the cord is tethered at that level. Spina bifida is almost always associated, and vertebral and sacral anomalies are found in as many as one-half of cases. MRI is the method of choice for evaluating LMMs as it is noninvasive and can demonstrate the full extent of the lipoma. Sagittal and axial T1-weighted images fully evaluate the relationship of the lipoma with the neural tissue.

References

1. Baker RA. Spinal cord tumors: intramedullary and intradural/extramedullary. In: Taveras JM, Ferrucci JT, eds. *Radiology: diagnosis-imaging-intervention,* vol. 3. Philadelphia: J. B. Lippincott, 1986, Ch. 110; pp. 1–12.
2. Barkovich AJ. Neoplasms of the spine. In: Barkovich AJ, ed. *Contemporary neuroimaging: pediatric neuroimaging,* vol. 1. New York: Raven Press, 1990;273–91.
3. Byrd SE. Radiologic evaluation of the pediatric spine. In: Poznanski AK, Kirkpatrick JA, eds. *Syllabus: a categorical course in diagnostic radiology, pediatric radiology.* Oak Brook, IL: RSNA, 1989;247–260.
4. Enzmann DR, De La Paz RL. Tumor. In: Enzmann DR, De La Paz RL, Rubin JB, eds. *Magnetic resonance of the spine.* St. Louis: C. V. Mosby, 1990;176–236.

Submitted by: Robert A. Breit, M.D., and Sharon E. Byrd, M.D., Children's Memorial Hospital and Northwestern University Medical School, Chicago, Illinois; Rosalind B. Dietrich, M.B., Ch.B., Senior Editor.

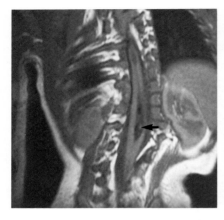

FIG. 42A. SE 550/20.

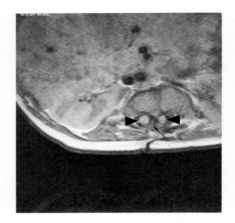

FIG. 42B. SE 1,000/20.

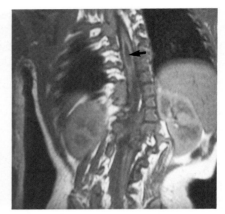

FIG. 42C. SE 550/20.

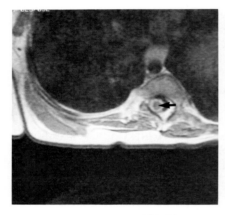

FIG. 42D. SE 1,000/20.

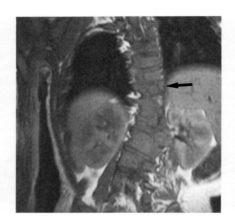

FIG. 42E. SE 550/20.

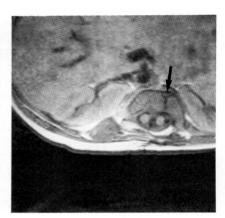

FIG. 42F. SE 1,000/20.

Clinical History

A child presented at birth with severe scoliosis and a lumbosacral hairy skin patch.

Findings

The coronal (SE 550/20) and axial (SE 1,000/20) images show the split spinal cord in the thoracolumbar region (Figs. 42A and B, *arrows*). It is difficult to determine the cephalad extent of the split on the coronal study (Figs. 42A and C). The axial images demonstrate the upper extent of the split and define an area of syringohydromyelia above the diastem (Figs. 42C and D, *arrows*). Note the scoliosis and multiple segmentation anomalies of the vertebrae (Figs. 42E and F).

Diagnosis

Diastematomyelia.

Discussion

Diastematomyelia refers to partial or complete clefting of the spinal cord, most common in the thoracic and lumbar levels. Pia surrounds each hemicord, each of which contains one ventral and one dorsal horn. Of patients with diastematomyelia, 60% have a single arachnoid and dural membrane surrounding the two hemicords. No bony spur or fibrous band is present in this form of diastematomyelia. The other 40% of patients have separate arachnoid and dural tubes surrounding each hemicord. Almost 100% of patients with this latter form of diastematomyelia have an associated fibrous band or bony spur passing between the hemicords.

Vertebral anomalies are almost always present, particularly spina bifida and fusion of the intersegmental laminae. Hemi-, butterfly, and block vertebrae are frequently observed. Kyphoscoliosis is present in the majority of patients.

Hydromyelia is seen in approximately one-half of patients and may involve one or both hemicords. Thickening of the filum terminale (greater than 2 mm) is commonly associated. Symptoms are generally seen in patients with fully duplicated meninges, and resection of the spur or band is necessary to relieve cord tethering.

MRI demonstrates the characteristic findings in diastematomyelia without the need for intrathecal contrast. Axial and coronal T1-weighted images are usually adequate to evaluate the clefting of the spinal cord. The ossified spur is seen as an area of signal void cortex extending between the two hemicords, although the center of the spur can present with varying degrees of hyperintensity should yellow marrow be present. MR easily demonstrates cord tethering and hydromyelia.

References

1. Barkovich AJ, Naidich TP. Congenital anomalies of the spine. In: Barkovich AJ, ed. *Contemporary neuroimaging: pediatric neuroimaging,* vol. 1. New York: Raven Press, 1990;227–271.
2. Byrd SE. Radiologic evaluation of the pediatric spine. In: Poznanski AK, Kirkpatrick JA, eds. *Syllabus: a categorical course in diagnostic radiology, pediatric radiology.* Oak Brook, IL: RSNA, 1989;247–260.
3. De La Paz RL. Congenital anomalies of the spine and spinal cord. In: Enzmann DR, De La Paz RL, Rubin JB, eds. *Magnetic resonance of the spine.* St. Louis: C. V. Mosby, 1990;176–236.
4. Naidich TP, McLone DG. Congential pathology of the spine and spinal cord. In: Taveras JM, Ferucci JT, eds. *Radiology: diagnosis-imaging-intervention,* vol. 3. Philadelphia: J. B. Lippincott, 1986, Ch. 103, pp. 1–23.

Submitted by: Robert A. Breit, M.D., and Sharon E. Byrd, M.D., Children's Memorial Hospital and Northwestern University Medical School, Chicago, Illinois; Rosalind B. Dietrich, M.B., Ch.B., Senior Editor.

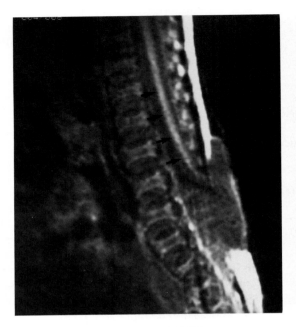

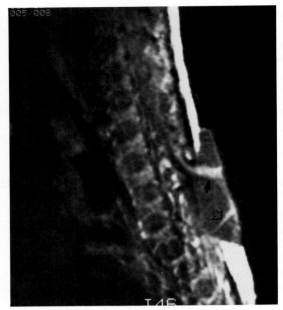

FIG. 43A. SE 600/30.

FIG. 43B. SE 600/30.

Clinical History

A 1-day-old infant was born with a midline lumbar back mass.

Findings

Sagittal (SE 600/30) images of the lower spine demonstrate tethering of the spinal cord to the back mass in the lumbar spine (Figs. 43A and B, *arrows*). The cord extends to an area of signal intensity similar to the cord itself (Fig. 43B, *arrowheads*). This area is superficially located with no overlying skin or fat. A nerve root extends forward from this tissue (Fig. 43B, *open arrow*). The CSF space is focally expanded and continuous into the mass.

Diagnosis

Myelomeningocele (MM).

Discussion

The term spinal dysraphism describes a group of malformations with incomplete fusion of midline mesenchymal, bony, and/or neural structures. There are three broad categories of spinal dysraphism: The first is associated with a back mass not covered by skin (MM, myelocele); the second is associated with a skin-covered mass (meningocele, lipomyelomeningocele, and myelocystocele); the third is the occult type, not associated with a back mass (diastematomyelia, intradural lipoma, dorsal dermal sinus, and tight filum terminale syndrome).

Both myeloceles and MMs are probably due to a localized abnormality in neural tube closure. The neural plate is initially continuous with the ectodermal skin. This primitive neural tissue normally separates from the ectoderm and folds into a tube. If separation fails, neural tube closure does not proceed and the neural tissue is exposed, remaining contiguous with the local skin. This neural tissue is called the neural placode, the exposed surface of which would normally form the ependymal lining of the central canal. The myelocele and MM are identical except that the placode of the myelocele is flush with the skin surface, whereas there is expansion of the subarachnoid space ventral to the placode in an MM, creating a sac that protrudes posterior to the skin surface. MMs are most commonly found in the lumbosacral spine, occasionally involving the thoracic spine. The spinal cord is always tethered to the placode. A midline bony defect is always present, whereas varying degrees of kyphoscoliosis are almost always present. All children with MM have Chiari II malformations of the hindbrain, and 40%–60% develop hydromyelia.

Imaging studies of the back are generally not performed in the newborn, as these children require urgent surgical treatment to close the defect. Because as many as 95% of patients with MM require ventricular shunting for hydrocephalus, ultrasound of the head is usually the only procedure necessary initially. The greatest role for MRI is following repair of the MM. Should a change in the child's neurologic status occur, the entire neural axis must be examined. The search is particularly for hydrocephalus, hydromyelia, and associated anomalies such as diastematomyelia (which occurs in approximately one-third of patients with MM), or for tethering of the cord at the repair site.

References

1. Barkovich AJ, Naidich TP. Congenital anomalies of the spine. In: Barkovich AJ, ed. *Contemporary neuroimaging: pediatric neuroimaging,* vol. 1. New York: Raven Press, 1990;227–271.
2. Byrd SE. Radiologic evaluation of the pediatric spine. In: Poznanski AK, Kirkpatrick JA, eds. *Syllabus: a categorical course in diagnostic radiology, pediatric radiology.* Oak Brook, IL: RSNA, 1989;247–260.
3. De La Paz RL. Congenital anomalies of the spine and spinal cord. In: Enzmann DR, De La Paz RL, Rubin JB, eds. *Magnetic resonance of the spine.* St. Louis: C. V. Mosby, 1990;176–236.
4. Naidich TP, McLone DG. Congenital pathology of the spine and spinal cord. In: Taveras JM, Ferucci JT, eds. *Radiology: diagnosis-imaging-intervention,* vol. 3. Philadelphia: J. B. Lippincott, 1986, Ch. 103, pp. 1–23.

Submitted by: Robert A. Breit, M.D., and Sharon E. Byrd, M.D., Children's Memorial Hospital and Northwestern University Medical School, Chicago, Illinois; Rosalind B. Dietrich, M.B., Ch.B., Senior Editor.

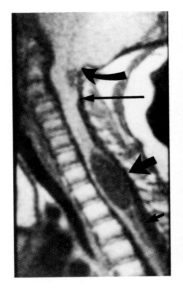 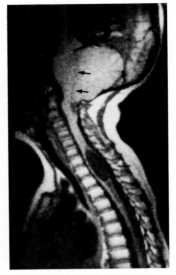

FIG. 44A. SE 500/30.   FIG. 44B. SE 500/30.

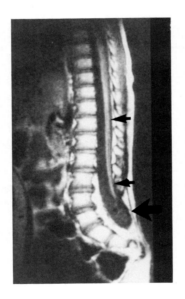

FIG. 44C. SE 500/30.

Clinical History

A 5-year-old girl with a new onset of hamstring spasticity.

Findings

Sagittal (SE 500/30) images of the spine demonstrate a somewhat eccentric cystic cavity in the cervicothoracic region of the spinal cord (Fig. 44A, *large arrow*). The cord is focally expanded and the caudal margin of the cavity is poorly defined (Fig. 44A, *small arrow*). The important "incidental" findings include cerebellar tonsilar herniation through the foramen magnum (Fig. 44A, *curved arrow*) and the cervicomedullary kink at C3–4 (Fig. 44A, *long arrow*). There are also narrowing and elongation of the fourth ventricle (Fig. 44B, *small arrows*) and tectal beaking (Fig. 44B, *curved arrow*). In the lumbosacral area the thecal sac is patulous, extending to the subcutaneous tissues (Fig. 44C, *large arrow*); the spinal cord is posteriorly positioned and extends to the dilated distal thecal sac (Fig. 44C, *small arrows*). There is questionable dilatation of the central canal in this portion of the cord.

Diagnosis

This is syringohydromyelia in a patient with Chiari II malformation. The changes in the lumbosacral region represent the postoperative appearance following the repair of a myelomeningocele.

Discussion

The term "syringohydromyelia" refers to a fluid cavity in the spinal cord, generally associated with gliosis. "Hydromyelia" is dilatation of the central canal, whereas the term "syringomyelia" is used for a cavity of the spinal cord that is removed from the central canal. As it is usually difficult to differentiate between these two entities, the term syringohydromyelia is usually appropriate.

Various theories for syringohydromyelia formation have been proposed, and their discussion is beyond the scope of this review. A good summary is presented in ref. 1. Syringohydromyelia is associated with Chiari I malformation, traumatic myelomalacia, spinal cord tumor, and arachnoiditis and is frequently idiopathic.

The method of choice for the evaluation of syringohydromyelia is MRI. In children, both 3 mm sagittal and 5 mm axial T1-weighted images are necessary to access the full extent of the cavity. On the T1-weighted images the cavity has CSF intensity, often demonstrating multiple septations. The caliber of the cord is usually enlarged by the cavity, but occasionally it is normal or decreased in size owing to pressure atrophy of the cord parenchyma. T2-weighted images may show an increased signal within the cord parenchyma at either end of the cavity. This is usually secondary to gliosis and should not enhance with contrast infusion.

Upon discovery of an area of syringohydromyelia an underlying cause must be searched for. The craniocervical junction should be examined for Chiari I malformation (cerebellar tonsils greater than 5 mm below the foramen magnum) and tumor. CSF loculations suggest previous arachnoid inflammation. Unless there is a history of prior cord trauma, patients who have syringohydromyelia should be studied with intravenous contrast to rule out a tumor. Occasionally, patients with Chiari I malformation and associated syrinx harbor underlying spinal cord tumors.

References

1. Barkovich AJ, Naidich TP. Congenital anomalies of the spine. In: Barkovich AJ, ed. *Contemporary neuroimaging: pediatric neuroimaging,* vol. 1. New York: Raven Press, 1990;227–271.
2. Byrd SE. Radiologic evaluation of the pediatric spine. In: Poznanski AK, Kirkpatrick JA, eds. *Syllabus: a categorical course in diagnostic radiology, pediatric radiology.* Oak Brook, IL: RSNA, 1989;247–260.
3. De La Paz RL. Congenital anomalies of the spine and spinal cord. In: Enzmann DR, De La Paz RL, Rubin JB. *Magnetic resonance of the spine.* St. Louis: C. V. Mosby, 1990;176–236.
4. Naidich TP, McLone DG. Congenital pathology of the spine and spinal cord. In: Taveras JM, Ferucci JT, eds. *Radiology: diagnosis-imaging-intervention,* vol. 3. Philadelphia: J. B. Lippincott, 1986, Ch. 103, pp. 1–23.

Submitted by: Robert A. Breit, M.D., and Sharon E. Byrd, M.D., Children's Memorial Hospital and Northwestern University Medical School, Chicago, Illinois; Rosalind B. Dietrich, M.B., Ch.B., Senior Editor.

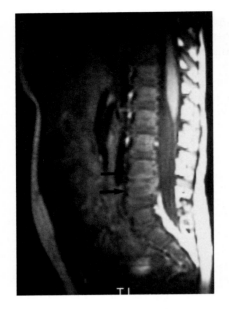
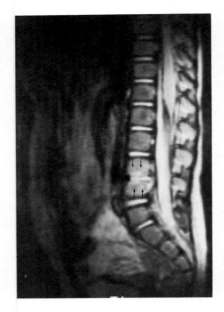
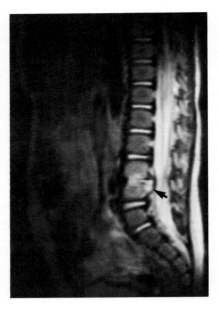

FIG. 45A. SE 650/20.   FIG. 45B. SE 2,000/80.   FIG. 45C. SE 2,000/80.

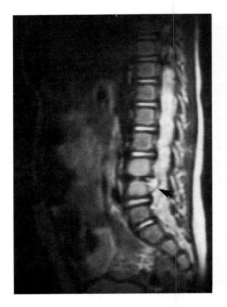
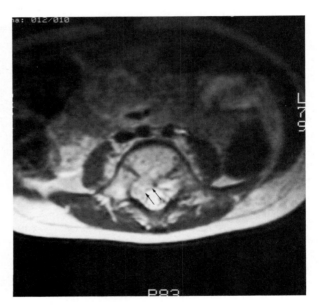

FIG. 45D. SE 2,000/80.   FIG. 45E. SE 2,000/80.

Clinical History

A 15-month-old child with a 1½-week history of an upper respiratory infection and fever who then presented with limping and refusal to walk. A bone scan demonstrated an abnormality at the L3–L4 disc level.

Findings

All sagittal sequences show loss of the endplates about the L4–5 intervertebral disc (Figs. 45A–D), as well as the obliteration of the normal disc anatomy. The signal intensity in the L4 and L5 vertebrae is low on the T1-weighted images (Fig. 45A, *arrows*) and bright on the T2-weighted images (Fig. 45B, *arrows*). There is epidural bright signal compromising the thecal sac ventrolaterally on the right (Figs. 45D and E, *arrows*), which represents either abscess or granulation tissue.

Diagnosis

Discitis.

Discussion

Intervertebral disc space infection is generally an extension of osteomyelitis of the subjacent vertebral body. Except in the instance of direct inoculation of the disc during an interventional or surgical procedure, this is considered the mode of progression in adults. A direct hematogenous route to the disc exists in children that allows disc infection without prior vertebral osteomyelitis so that, in children, the term "discitis" is appropriate. Prior ear infection or upper respiratory infection is frequently an antecedent event. Although organisms are rarely isolated in childhood discitis, pyogenic organisms are generally presumed.

MR is the best overall imaging modality to evaluate discitis. Its sensitivity rivals radionuclide scans in the detection of this process; in addition MR allows for evaluation of the extent of spread of infection. MR reflects the inflammatory changes in the disc and bone marrow, disc space narrowing, and extension of inflammation into the surrounding soft tissues, including the epidural space. Inflammatory tissue is low in signal on T1-weighted images, and this is generally easily appreciated in adults; however, in young children, the axial skeletal marrow signal is also low and the inflammatory changes are not as easily detected. Involved vertebral body signal intensity is abnormally bright on T2-weighted images. The disc space narrowing can be appreciated on any sagittal sequence, and the signal intensity of the disc is usually bright on T2-weighted images, although occasionally it is iso- or hypointense relative to normal discs. Compromise of the spinal canal can occur secondary to granulation tissue or abscess within the anterior subligamentous or epidural space. Cortical margins of the vertebral body become obscured due to bony destruction.

References

1. Enzmann DR. Infection and inflammation. In: Enzmann DR, De La Paz RL, Rubin JB, eds. *Magnetic resonance of the spine.* St. Louis: C. V. Mosby, 1990;260–300.
2. Resnick D, Niwayama G. Osteomyelitis, septic arthritis, and soft tissue infection: the axial skeleton. In: Resnick D, Niwayama G, eds. *Diagnosis of bone and joint disorders.* Philadelphia: W. B. Saunders, 1981;2130–2153.
3. Resnick D, Niwayama G. Osteomyelitis, septic arthritis, and soft tissue infection: organisms. In: Resnick D, Niwayama G, eds. *Diagnosis of bone and joint disorders.* Philadelphia: W. B. Saunders, 1981;2154–2237.
4. Wenger DR, Bobechko WP. Spectrum of intervertebral disc-space infection in children. *Bone Joint Surg* 1978;60:100–108.

Submitted by: Robert A. Breit, M.D., and Sharon E. Byrd, M.D., Children's Memorial Hospital and Northwestern University Medical School, Chicago, Illinois; Rosalind B. Dietrich, M.B., Ch.B., Senior Editor.

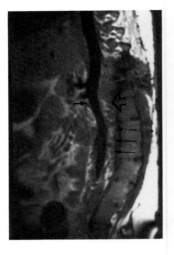

FIG. 46A. SE 733/20.

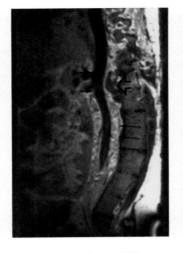

FIG. 46B. SE 717/30 with Gd-DTPA.

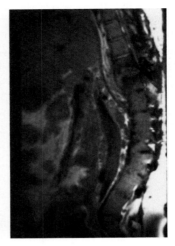

FIG. 46C. SE 733/20.

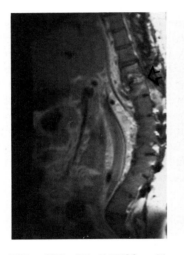

FIG. 46D. SE 717/20 with Gd-DTPA.

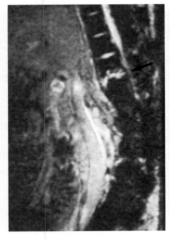

FIG. 46E. SE 500/30 with Gd-DTPA.

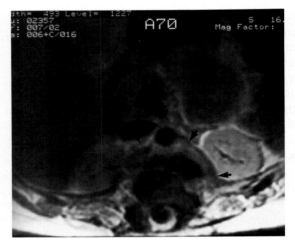

FIG. 46F. SE 800/20 with Gd-DTPA.

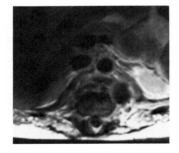

FIG. 46G. SE 800/30 with Gd-DTPA.

Clinical History

A 15-year-old female with status/post-myelomeningocele repair, ventriculo-peritoneal shunt, and multiple orthopedic procedures for severe scoliosis. The patient has had 2 weeks of fever, back pain, and a positive gallium scan in the thoracolumbar spine.

Findings

The patient is severely scoliotic. The sagittal T1-weighted images of the thoracolumbar spine demonstrate a mottled intensity expansion of the prevertebral tissues (Fig. 46A, *long arrows* and *open arrow*) with forward bowing of the aorta by mass effect (Fig. 46A, *short arrows*). Post-infusion T1-weighted sagittal images show intense enhancement of the prevertebral tissues (Fig. 46B, *long arrows*) with irregular loculations of fluid (Fig. 46B, *open arrow*). The pre- (Fig. 46C) and post-gadolinium-DTPA (Fig. 46D) sagittal T1-weighted images show lower thoracic enhancing inflammatory tissue centered at the disc level with obliteration of the normal disc anatomy (*open arrow*). Notice that the low signal in the adjacent vertebrae enhances and the adjacent endplates are destroyed. (See also Fig. 46E, *arrow*). The axial images show the displacement of the IVC and aorta by the inflammatory mass (Fig. 46F, *arrows*).

Diagnosis

Infectious spondylitis with paraspinal abscess.

Discussion

Infections of the spine occur hematogenously via the arterial or Batson's venous plexus route. Alternatively, infection is due to direct inoculation following surgery or any type of spinal needle puncture. The most common causative organism is *Staphylococcus aureus.* Pain and fever are the usual clinical findings, whereas paraparesis is only rarely observed late in the course of disease. Infections of the spine are more frequent in adults than in children. In children, a direct hematogenous route to the disc itself exists that allows disc space infection without prior vertebral osteomyelitis, so that, in children, the term "discitis" may occasionally be appropriate.

The organism usually seeds the subchondral space of the vertebral body anteriorly. The infection can then spread to the adjacent vertebrae by the following routes: (a) through the disc and (b) into the subligamentous space deep to the anterior longitudinal ligament (ALL). The paraspinal tissues can be involved once the ALL has been breached. Generally, two adjacent vertebrae plus the disc space bridging them are involved. It is rare to see involvement of the posterior elements.

MR is the best overall imaging modality to evaluate infectious spondylitis. Its sensitivity rivals radionuclide scans in the detection of this process; in addition, MR allows for evaluation of the extent of spread of infection. MR reflects the inflammatory changes in the disc and bone marrow, disc space narrowing, and extension of inflammation into the surrounding soft tissues, including the epidural space. Inflammatory tissue is low in signal on T1-weighted images, and this is generally easily appreciated in adults; however, in young children, the axial skeletal marrow signal is also low and the inflammatory changes are not as easily detected. Involved vertebral body signal intensity is abnormally bright on T2-weighted images. The disc space narrowing can be appreciated on any sagittal sequence and the signal intensity of the disc is usually bright on T2-weighted images, although occasionally it is iso- or hypointense relative to normal discs. Compromise of the spinal canal can occur secondary to granulation tissue or abscess within the posterior subligamentous or epidural space. Cortical margins of the vertebral body become obscured due to bony destruction.

References

1. Enzmann DR. Infection and inflammation. In: Enzmann DR, De La Paz RL, Rubin JB, eds. *Magnetic resonance of the spine.* St. Louis: C. V. Mosby, 1990;260–300.
2. Resnick D, Niwayama G. Osteomyelitis, septic arthritis, and soft tissue infection: the axial skeleton. In: Resnick D, Niwayama G, eds. *Diagnosis of bone and joint disorders.* Philadelphia: W. B. Saunders, 1981;2130–2153.
3. Resnick D, Niwayama G. Osteomyelitis, septic arthritis, and soft tissue infection: organisms. In: Resnick D, Niwayama G, eds. *Diagnosis of bone and joint disorders.* Philadelphia: W. B. Saunders, 1981;2154–2237.
4. Wenger DR, Bobechko WP. Spectrum of intervertebral disc-space infection in children. *J Bone Joint Surg* 1978;60:100–108.

Submitted by: Robert A. Breit, M.D., and Sharon E. Byrd, M.D., Children's Memorial Hospital and Northwestern University Medical School, Chicago, Illinois; Rosalind B. Dietrich, M.B., Ch.B., Senior Editor.

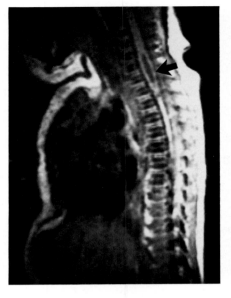

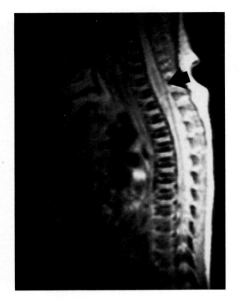

FIG. 47A. SE 600/20.

FIG. 47B. SE 2,022/30.

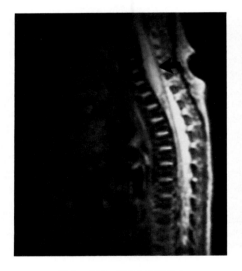

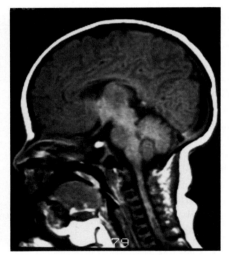

FIG. 47C. SE 2,022/80.

FIG. 47D. SE 600/20.

Clinical History

An infant was noted to be paraplegic at 2 weeks of age.

Findings

The sagittal MR (SE 600/30) image demonstrates a focal enlargement of the cervicothoracic spinal cord due to a cystic cavity (Fig. 47A, *arrow*), the signal intensity of which becomes increasingly brighter with increasing T2 weighting on the (SE 2,022/30) and (SE 2,022/80) images (Figs. 47B and C, *arrows*). There is no spinal cord mass above or below the cavity. Post-contrast images (not shown) show no pathologic enhancement. No Chiari I malformation is present (Fig. 47D).

Diagnosis

Syringohydromyelia secondary to a cervicothoracic astrocytoma diagnosed by biopsy.

Discussion

In the pediatric population astrocytoma accounts for approximately 60% of intramedullary tumors, whereas ependymoma accounts for 30%. This is roughly the reverse of the incidence noted in adults. The most common location for astrocytoma is the cervical or cervicothoracic cord followed by the conus medullaris. Although all age groups are affected, the highest incidence is in children approximately 10 years old.

At the level of the neoplasm the cord is enlarged. Usually only a small number of cord segments is involved by tumor, but the extent of cord enlargement is frequently altered by the presence of cysts above or below the tumor. Associated cysts are present in as many as 40% of cases. Occasionally the tumor can involve a large number of cord segments.

MRI is the method of choice for evaluating the patient suspected of harboring a spinal cord neoplasm and in following a known lesion. T2-weighted images demonstrate the cord enlargement and the tumor is usually bright, but the tumor itself cannot be confidently differentiated from tumor necrosis or cystic cavities. This is accomplished with T1-weighted images and gadolinium-DTPA. A cystic cavity or area of necrosis will remain relatively low in signal intensity on T1-weighted images, whereas the solid portion of the tumor exhibits intense enhancement, thus allowing for a clear distinction to be made. Two caveats are necessary with regard to tumoral enhancement. First, the tumor margins generally extend beyond the margin of enhancement (although not to the same degree as in the brain); second, not all astrocytomas enhance.

In any patient without a history of cord trauma or Chiari I in whom a cystic cavity (syringohydromyelia) is discovered, administration of intravenous contrast is necessary to rule out an underlying tumor. Once the tumor is discovered, it is not necessary to differentiate between astrocytoma and ependymoma as the treatment will not differ.

References

1. Baker RA. Spinal cord tumors: intramedullary and intradural/extramedullary. In: Taveras JM, Ferrucci JT, eds. *Radiology: diagnosis-imaging-intervention,* vol. 3. Philadelphia: J. B. Lippincott, 1986, Ch. 110, pp. 1–12.
2. Barkovich AJ. Neoplasms of the spine. In: Barkovich AJ, ed. *Contemporary neuroimaging: pediatric neuroimaging,* vol. 1. New York: Raven Press, 1990;273–291.
3. Byrd SE. Radiologic evaluation of the pediatric spine. In: Poznanski AK, Kirkpatrick JA, eds. *Syllabus: a categorical course in diagnostic radiology, pediatric radiology.* Oak Brook, IL: RSNA, 1989;247–260.
4. Enzmann DR, De La Paz RL. Tumor. In: Enzmann DR, De La Paz RL, Rubin JB, eds. *Magnetic resonance of the spine.* St. Louis: C. V. Mosby, 1990;176–236.

Submitted by: Robert A. Breit, M.D., and Sharon E. Byrd, M.D., Children's Memorial Hospital and Northwestern University Medical School, Chicago, Illinois; Rosalind B. Dietrich, M.B., Ch.B., Senior Editor.

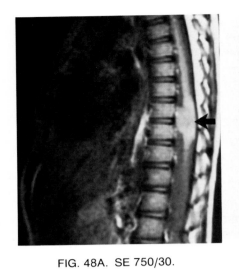

FIG. 48A. SE 750/30.

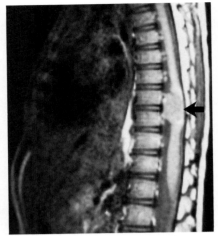

FIG. 48B. SE 750/30.

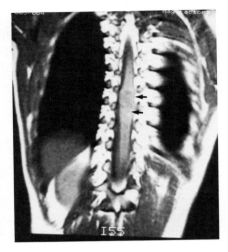

FIG. 48C. SE 733/30.

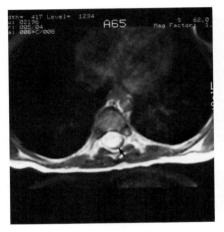

FIG. 48D. SE 800/30 with Gd-DTPA.

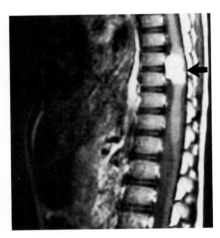

FIG. 48E. SE 750/30 with Gd-DTPA.

Clinical History

A 3-year-old boy presented with a 6-week history of a bilateral lower extremity weakness along with right lower extremity hypertonia and a positive Babinski sign.

Findings

Sagittal and coronal MR (SE 750/30) images demonstrate a focal enlargement of the spinal cord with ill-defined margins; the signal intensity of the lesion is slightly less than that of the cord (Figs. 48A–C, *arrows*). The post-contrast T1-weighted spin-echo axial and sagittal images show intense homogeneous enhancement (Figs. 48D and E, *arrows*). The tumor replaces and compresses normal cord and exhibits exophytic growth.

Diagnosis

Spinal cord ependymoma.

Discussion

In the pediatric age population the two most common intramedullary tumors are astrocytoma and ependymoma. Ependymoma accounts for approximately 30% of these, whereas the majority of spinal cord tumors are astrocytomas. The reverse of this incidence is observed in the adult population. The most common location for ependymoma is the conus medullaris, followed by the cervical and cervicothoracic regions. Astrocytomas are more frequently located more rostrally. At the level of the neoplasm the cord is generally enlarged. Usually only a small number of cord segments is involved by tumor, but the extent of cord enlargement is frequently altered by the presence of cysts above or below the tumor. Associated cysts are present in as many as 40% of cases. Occasionally the tumor can involve a large number of cord segments.

MRI is the method of choice for evaluating the patient suspected of harboring a spinal cord neoplasm and in following a known lesion. With the use of intravenous paramagnetic contrast infusion only T1-weighted imaging is necessary. The T2-weighted images demonstrate cord enlargement and the tumor is usually bright, but the tumor cannot be confidently differentiated from tumor necrosis or cystic cavities. This is accomplished with contrast infusion. A cystic cavity or area of necrosis will remain relatively low signal intensity on T1-weighted images, whereas the solid portion of tumor exhibits intense enhancement, thus allowing for a clear distinction to be made. Two caveats are necessary with regard to tumoral enhancement. First, the tumor generally extends beyond the margin of enhancement; second, not all intramedullary tumors enhance.

In any patient without a history of cord trauma in whom a cystic cavity (syringohydromyelia) is discovered, administration of intravenous contrast is necessary to rule out an underlying tumor. Once the tumor is discovered, it is not necessary nor is it possible to differentiate between astrocytoma and ependymoma, as this distinction will not alter the therapy.

References

1. Baker RA. Spinal cord tumors: intramedullary and intradural/extramedullary. In: Taveras JM, Ferrucci JT, eds. *Radiology: diagnosis-imaging-intervention,* vol. 3. Philadelphia: J. B. Lippincott, 1986 Ch. 110, pp. 1–12.
2. Barkovich AJ. Neoplasms of the spine. In: Barkovich AJ, ed. *Contemporary neuroimaging: pediatric neuroimaging,* vol. 1. New York: Raven Press, 1990;273–291.
3. Byrd SE. Radiologic evaluation of the pediatric spine. In: Poznanski AK, Kirkpatrick JA, eds. *Syllabus: a categorical course in diagnostic radiology, pediatric radiology.* Oak Brook, IL: RSNA, 1989;247–260.
4. Enzmann DR, De La Paz RL. Tumor. In: Enzmann DR, De La Paz RL, Rubin JB, eds. *Magnetic resonance of the spine.* St. Louis: C. V. Mosby, 1990;176–236.

Submitted by: Robert A. Breit, M.D., and Sharon E. Byrd, M.D., Children's Memorial Hospital and Northwestern University Medical School, Chicago, Illinois; Rosalind B. Dietrich, M.B., Ch.B., Senior Editor.

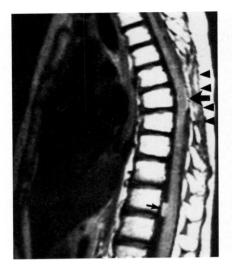

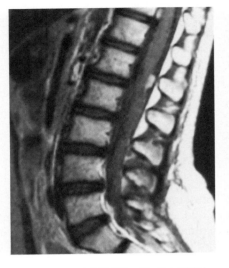

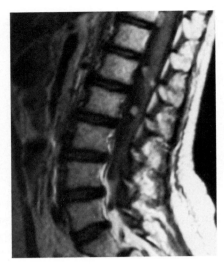

FIG. 49A. SE 500/30 with Gd-DTPA.　　FIG. 49B. SE 500/30 with Gd-DTPA.　　FIG. 49C. SE 500/30 with Gd-DTPA.

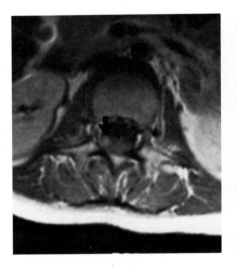

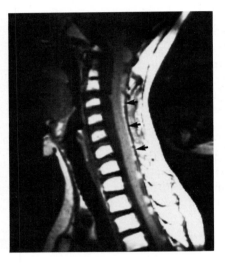

FIG. 49D. SE 800/20 with Gd-DTPA.　　FIG. 49E. SE 600/20 with Gd-DTPA.

Clinical History

A 10-year-old-girl who had presented 6 months prior to this MR study with a history of back pain and progressive lower extremity weakness.

Findings

In these post-contrast T1-weighted sagittal images, there is an enhancing nodule (Fig. 49A, *small arrow*) along with postoperative changes characterized by the missing posterior elements (Fig. 49A, *arrowheads*) in the mid-thoracic region and adherence of the cord posteriorly (Fig. 49A, *large arrow*). Notice the bright signal in all of the vertebral bodies indicating fatty marrow secondary to previous irradiation (Figs. 49A and E). Multiple enhancing nodules lie along the spinal cord and roots of the cauda equina (Figs. 49B–E) along with "coating" of the cervical cord by enhancing tumor (Fig. 49E).

Diagnosis

Drop metastases secondary to a fourth ventricular ependymoma.

Discussion

The term "drop metastasis" refers to the CSF spread into the spinal canal of a primary CNS tumor. This mode of metastasis is observed more frequently in the pediatric population than in adults. The common neoplasms to spread by this route include medulloblastoma, high-grade glioma, ependymoma, germinoma, and pineal gland tumors. Medulloblastoma is by far the most frequent tumor to seed the CSF, particularly in the spine, and does so in one-third of patients. The better differentiated medulloblastomas paradoxically spread by the CSF route with greater frequency than the more histologically malignant tumors.

Ependymomas rarely present initially with spinal drop metastases but generally present at the time of local recurrence, especially fourth ventricular primary tumors. Drop metastases are most commonly observed in the thoracic and lumbosacral regions. Myelography and postmyelography CT demonstrate nodular filling defects and irregularity and clumping of nerve roots. Cytology can be accomplished simultaneously.

T1-weighted images may show tumor nodules along the cord or nerve roots of the cauda equina but may only show clumping and adherence of nerve roots, thus mimicking arachnoiditis. The high signal intensity of the tumor on T2-weighted images is often obscured by the surrounding bright CSF signal. Clearly, small tumors and tumors coating the spinal cord or nerve roots can be easily missed by myelography, CT myelography, and conventional T1- and T2-weighted images. Routine use of intravenous contrast with T1-weighted images is necessary to correctly detect leptomeningeal spread of tumor. Intense enhancement of tumor nodules is easy to detect. One may see a thin line of enhancement along the spinal cord or nerve roots when sheets of tumor cells coat these structures.

In children it is rare for other primary tumors to metastasize to the meninges by non-CSF spread. An important exception is the leukemias and lymphomas, which tend to infiltrate the meninges. In these patients and in all patients suspected of having drop metastases, T1-weighted post-infusion imaging is the method of choice.

References

1. Baker RA. Spinal cord tumors: intramedullary and intradural/extramedullary. In: Taveras JM, Ferrucci JT, eds. *Radiology: diagnosis-imaging-intervention,* vol. 3. Philadelphia: J. B. Lippincott, 1986, Ch. 110, pp. 1–12.
2. Barkovich AJ. Neoplasms of the spine. In: Barkovich AJ, ed. *Contemporary neuroimaging: pediatric neuroimaging,* vol. 1. New York: Raven Press, 1990;273–291.
3. Byrd SE. Radiologic evaluation of the pediatric spine. In: Poznanski AK, Kirkpatrick JA, eds. *Syllabus: a categorical course in diagnostic radiology, pediatric radiology.* Oak Brook, IL: RSNA, 1989;247–260.
4. Enzmann DR, De La Paz RL. Tumor. In: Enzmann DR, De La Paz RL, Rubin JB, eds. *Magnetic resonance of the spine.* St. Louis: C. V. Mosby, 1990;176–236.

Submitted by: Robert A. Breit, M.D., and Sharon E. Byrd, M.D., Children's Memorial Hospital and Northwestern University Medical School, Chicago, Illinois; Rosalind B. Dietrich, M.B., Ch.B., Senior Editor.

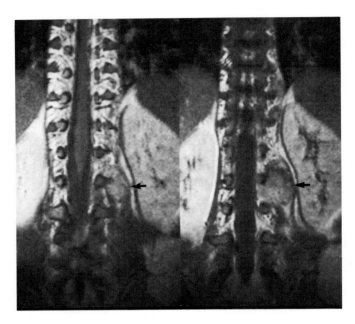

FIG. 50A. SE 600/20.

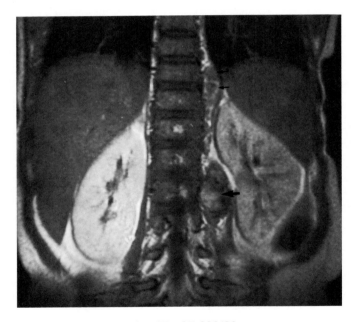

FIG. 50B. SE 600/20.

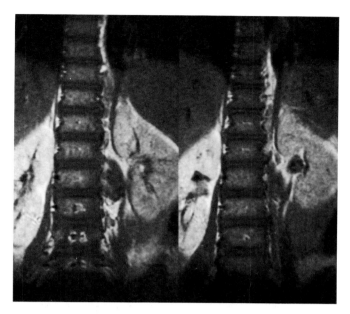

FIG. 50C. SE 600/20.

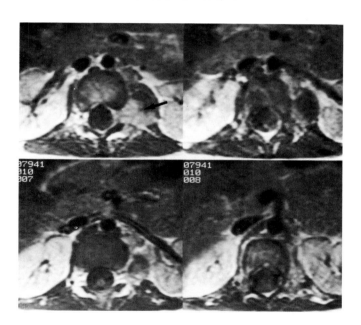

FIG. 50D. SE 600/20.

117

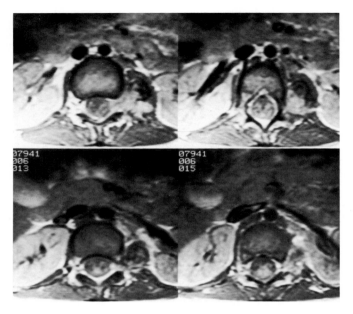

FIG. 50E. SE 600/20.

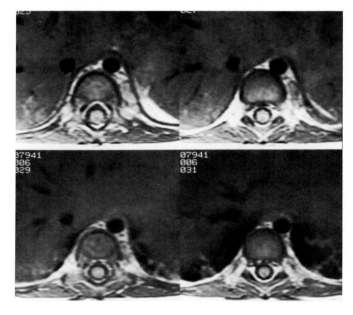

FIG. 50F. SE 600/20.

Clinical History

A 2-year-old girl was admitted to the hospital with opsoclonus, myoclonus syndrome, and ataxia. She was unable to walk unassisted.

Findings

MR images demonstrate a left paravertebral multi-lobulated retroperitoneal soft tissue mass (Figs. 50A–C, *black arrows*). It extends from T9 through L4, (Fig. 50B, *small black arrows*) with a globular component of the mass lying in the hilum of the kidney (Fig. 50A). The kidney is seen to be displaced laterally. At L1–2 and L2–3 the tumor extends through the neural foramina into the epidural space (Figs. 50D and E, *black arrows*). Superiorly, the tumor displaces the left crus of the diaphragm (Fig. 50F).

Diagnosis

Neuroblastoma.

Discussion

Neuroblastoma is the most common solid abdominal neoplasm in childhood. Neuroblastomas arise from ganglion cells, in the sympathetic chain or para-aortic bodies and in the adrenal glands. The most common location is in the abdomen, where it most frequently arises from the adrenals (1).

MRI is helpful in demonstrating the site and size of the mass, and when a diagnosis has been established, in staging the lesion.

T1-weighted images demonstrate anatomy, distinguish adrenal from renal and hepatic tissue, and demonstrate any intraspinal extension (2).

Vascular anatomy is also well demonstrated and of importance for evaluating tumor resectability (1). The tumor often extends across the midline and may encase vessels. The aorta and inferior vena cava are usually very well shown on coronal T1-weighted scans. The origins of the celiac axis and superior mesenteric artery are better seen on transverse or sagittal images (1).

MRI can also be used to demonstrate metastases to liver, bone, bone marrow, and dura (3,4).

When neuroblastoma is located in the paraspinal region, local extension into the spinal canal can occur. Approximately 14% of patients with neuroblastoma or ganglioneuroblastoma have intraspinal extension (2).

Preoperative diagnosis of intraspinal extension is important for treatment planning. MRI is noninvasive, and this is an advantage over CT with metrizamide myelography, which was formerly used.

MRI shows the interface between tumor and spinal contents because of difference in signal intensity between CSF and soft tissues (2).

References

1. Dietrich RB, Kangarloo H. Pediatric body imaging. In: Bradley WG, Stark DC, eds. *Magnetic resonance imaging.* St. Louis: C. V. Mosby, 1988, pp. 1434–1453.
2. Siegel MJ, Jamroz GA, Glazer HS, Abramson CL. MR imaging of intraspinal extension of neuroblastoma. *J Comput Assist Tomogr* 1986;10:593–595.
3. Dietrich RB, Kangarloo H, Lenarsky C, et al. Neuroblastoma: the role of magnetic resonance imaging. *AJR* 1987;148:937.
4. Dietrich RB, Kangarloo M. Diagnostic oncology case study. Retroperitoneal mass with intradural extension: value of magnetic resonance imaging in neuroblastoma. *AJR* 1986;146:251.

Submitted by: Patricia E. Perry, M.D., Good Samaritan Regional Medical Center and Phoenix Children's Hospital, Phoenix, Arizona; Rosalind B. Dietrich, M.B., Ch.B., Senior Editor.

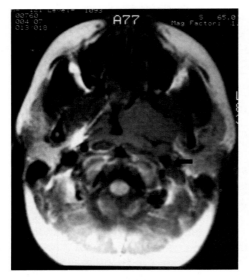

FIG. 51A. SE 800/20.

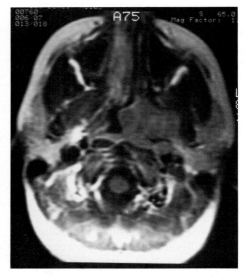

FIG. 51B. SE 400/20 with Gd-DTPA.

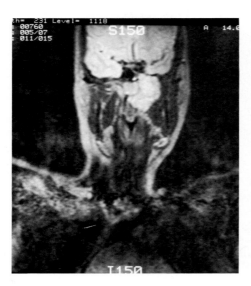

FIG. 51C. SE 2,000/80.

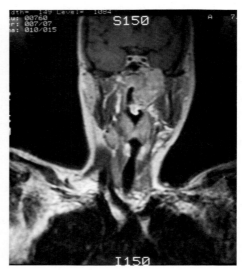

FIG. 51D. SE 700/20.

Clinical History

A 19-year-old white female presented with nasal congestion. The patient has a history of a tumor removed from her neck 1 year prior to her current presentation.

Findings

There is a 4 × 5 cm solid mass in the left parapharyngeal space lying medial to the parapharyngeal fat (Fig. 51A). The mass displaces the parapharyngeal fat and medial pterygoid muscle laterally (Fig. 51A, *small arrows*) and the carotid sheath posteriorly (Fig. 51A, *large arrow*). The medial aspect of the mass protrudes into the nasopharyngeal airway. The signal intensity of the mass is intermediate between muscle and fat on T1-weighted images and hyperintense compared to muscle and fat on T2-weighted images (Fig. 51C). The mass shows slight enhancement on gadolinium-DTPA enhanced images (Fig. 51B).

The coronal images demonstrate asymmetry of the floor of the middle cranial fossa secondary to temporal lobe elevation by the tumor mass (Fig. 51D). The left sternocleidomastoid has been previously resected. No extension into the cavernous sinus is seen.

Diagnosis

Rhabdomyosarcoma, embryonal type.

Discussion

Rhabdomyosarcoma is the most common soft tissue tumor in children, adolescents, and young adults. In several studies, it represents almost 20% of all soft tissue tumors. Histologic classification identifies four categories: embryonal, botryoid, alveolar, and pleomorphic.

The embryonal type is the most common and accounts for 70%–80% of all rhabdomyosarcomas. The peak age of onset is from birth to 15 years. The botryoid type is a polypoid grape-like variant of the embryonal type. Most commonly it originates in mucosal-lined organs such as the vagina or urinary bladder.

Alveolar rhabdomyosarcoma represents 10%–20% of all rhabdomyosarcomas. It has a greater distribution in the extremities. The pleomorphic type is the rarest form and has a peak onset after age 45, affecting primarily the large muscles of the thigh.

The three most common locations for rhabdomyosarcoma are (a) head and neck (which account for 44% of occurrences), (b) genitourinary and retroperitoneal areas (accounting for 34% of cases), and (c) extremities (which represent almost 15% of occurrences).

The majority of the rhabdomyosarcomas arising in the nasopharynx are the embryonal type. Skull base invasion is common with extension into the cavernous sinus resulting in cranial nerve palsies. Local extension into the adjacent lymph nodes is seen in approximately one-half of cases. The lungs and bones are common sites of metastases. On MR, the lesion is usually bulky with signal intensity between that of muscle and fat on T1-weighted images. Evaluation of skull base extension is best performed by MR.

References

1. Madewell JE, Sweet DE. Tumors and tumor-like lesions in or about joints. In: Resnick D, Niwayama G, eds. *Diagnosis of bone and joint disorders.* Philadelphia: W. B. Saunders, 1981;2690–2751.
2. Enzinger FM, Weiss SW. *Soft tissue tumors,* 2nd ed. St. Louis: C. V. Mosby, 1988;448–488.
3. Cross RR, Shapiro MD, Som PM. MRI of the parapharyngeal space. *Radiol Clin North Am* 1989;27:353–378.

Submitted by: Jon Karstetter, M.D., and Yutaka Sato, M.D., University of Iowa Hospitals and Clinics, Iowa City, Iowa; Rosalind B. Dietrich, M.B., Ch.B., Senior Editor.

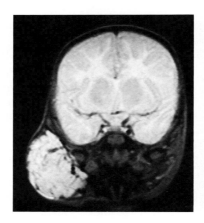 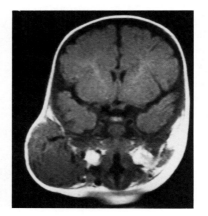

FIG. 52A. SE 2,000/100.   FIG. 52B. SE 583/20.

Clinical History

A newborn female with nontender, soft, right cheek mass without inflammation that has been present since birth. All lab values are within normal limits.

Findings

A large, 5 × 6 × 10 cm, mass with inhomogeneous signal located over the right mandible in the masticator space. This mass shows predominately intermediate signal intensity on T1-weighted images and hyperintense signal on T2-weighted images, but the internal signal characteristic is inhomogeneous on both T1- and T2-weighted images. The right retromandibular vein (Fig. 52A, *arrow*) and other dilated vascular structures are visualized as areas of tubular signal void (Figs. 52A and B). The right parotid gland is displaced posteriorly (Fig. 52A, *arrowhead*).

Diagnosis

Cavernous hemangioma of the right cheek.

Discussion

Vascular malformations occur as a result of arrested or maldevelopment of the vascular system. Vascular malformations can be categorized histologically into three types: capillary hemangiomas, arteriovenous malformations, and cavernous hemangiomas. There are microscopic communications at the capillary level in capillary hemangiomas. Angiography shows no evidence of arteriovenous shunting, but a dense stain or blush may be demonstrated. Arteriovenous malformations are characterized by a network of communications between arteries and veins with angiography revealing a variable amount of arteriovenous shunting. This shunting may be hemodynamically significant, occasionally resulting in high output congestive heart failure. Cavernous hemangiomas, on the other hand, contain tortuous, large, superficial veins. Angiographically there is no evidence of arteriovenous shunting.

Due to the high protein density and slow flow of blood, cavernous hemangiomas display high intensity signal on T2-weighted images. Coronal and sagittal images are helpful for assessment of the lesion's relationship to the surrounding tissues. This is important prior to treatment, either by surgery or embolectomy.

Thrombocytopenia may occur as a result of excessive consumption of circulating platelets on the damaged subendothelial surface of the neoplasm (Kasabach-Merritt syndrome).

The differential diagnosis for this lesion would include juvenile (or "strawberry") hemangioma. This is a type of capillary hemangioma that occurs in the skin of newborns. These vascular malformations grow rapidly in the first few months of life, begin to regress from 1 to 3 years of age, and resolve by age 5 in 80% of cases.

References

1. Itoh K, Nishimura K, Togoshi K, et al. Magnetic resonance imaging of cavernous hemangiomas of the face and neck. *J Comput Assist Tomogr* 1986;10:831–835.
2. Som PM, Braun IF, Shapiro MD, et al. Tumors of the parapharyngeal space and upper neck: magnetic resonance imaging characteristics. *Radiology* 1987;164:823–829.
3. MacCallum DW, Martin LW. Hemangioma in infancy and childhood. A report based in 6,479 cases. *Surg Clin North Am* 1957;36:1647.

Submitted by: Mark F. Rich, M.D., and Y. Sato, M.D., University of Iowa Hospitals and Clinics, Iowa City, Iowa; Rosalind B. Dietrich, M.B., Ch.B., Senior Editor.

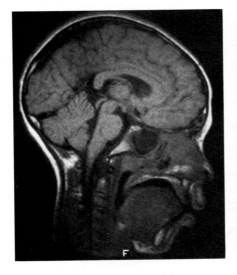

FIG. 53A. SE 466/26.

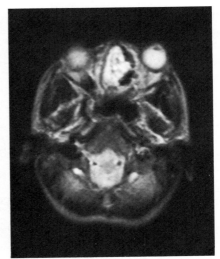

FIG. 53B. SE 1,800/100.

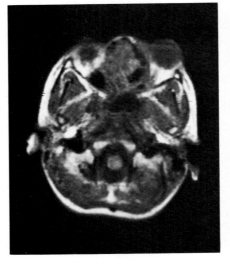

FIG. 53C. SE 633/26.

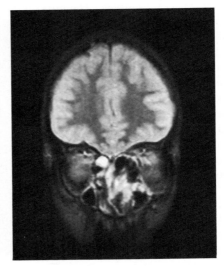

FIG. 53D. SE 1,800/100.

Clinical History

A previously healthy 11-year-old black male presented with a 1-week history of left eye proptosis and a 6-week history of nasal stuffiness and increased lacrimation from the left eye.

Findings

An enlarged sphenoid sinus of very low signal intensity is seen on T1-weighted sagittal and axial images (Fig. 53A, C). It is associated with a large, inhomogeneous mass that involves the ethmoid sinuses and extends into the left maxillary sinus. Extraconal involvement of the left orbit is seen on axial T2-weighted images. Figure 53B shows the impressively low attenuation signal in the sphenoid sinus as contrasted with the inhomogeneous but predominantly high signal seen in the ethmoid area and orbit. This finding is unusual but is a characteristic appearance of fungal sinusitis on T2-weighted images. These findings are thought to be due to the increased concentrations of iron and manganese present in mycetoma and the presence of calcium in the fungal concretions. Note the bony expansion, erosion, and destruction seen on the T2-weighted coronal images (Fig. 53D).

Diagnosis

Aspergillus fumigatus giant mucopyocele involving the ethmoid, frontal, left maxillary, and sphenoid sinuses.

Discussion

Aspergillus is a ubiquitous mold found in agricultural dusts that can cause severe infection in debilitated patients or diabetics, or as the result of alterations in the normal flora balance secondary to antibiotic use. It does occur in otherwise normal individuals, however, as in this instance.

Mucoceles result from chronic obstruction of a sinus ostium. Increased pressure secondary to continued mucous secretion causes sinus expansion and thinning of the bony sinus walls. Mucopyoceles frequently occur and can be caused by bacteria (common) or fungus.

Clinical signs and symptoms include proptosis, pain, increased lacrimation, headache, vertical diplopia, and orbital mass.

Radiographic findings on plain films are sinus opacity, with or without thinning and expansion of bony walls. Aggressive mucopyoceles can cause bone destruction (esp. lamina papyracea) and mimic malignancy. CT exams ordinarily reveal homogeneous and average density lesions; eventual drying of secretions in chronically obstructed sinuses results in mixed attenuation.

MR findings in typical bacterial sinusitis or mucopyoceles are long T1 and T2 relaxation times, thus high signal intensity, reflecting their increased water content.

However, fungal infections have been associated with combinations of short and long T1 and T2 relaxation times. Correlating gross viscosity of surgical specimens, macromolecular protein concentrations, amount of free water, and the concentrations of iron, manganese, and calcium between bacterial and fungal infectious processes, several interesting trends were seen.

These factors were found responsible for the inhomogeneous signal intensity of fungally infected sinuses on MR versus uniform attenuation on CT. Of particular interest was the very low signal seen on T1- and T2-weighted MR images in mycetomas, of which *aspergillis* is quite common. Increased concentrations of iron and manganese in mycetoma versus bacterially infected mucus and the higher calcium content in fungal concretions seem to be the major factors in play. These findings should raise the suspicion that fungal, not bacterial, sinus disease is the cause of the patient's illness, a major factor in appropriate therapy.

Differential diagnosis includes mucormycosis, clinically similar to, but much more aggressive than, *Aspergillis;* polyposis, usually secondary to chronic allergy; tumor, Lymphoma, esthesioneuroblastoma, juvenile angiofibroma.

References

1. Dodd GD, et al. Radiology of the nose, paranasal sinuses and nasopharynx. Section 2, 1977.
2. Hasso AN. CT of tumors and tumor-like conditions of the paranasal sinuses. *Radiol Clin North Am* 1984;22.
3. Hesselink JR, Weber AL. Infections of the sinuses and face. *Textbook of diagnostic imaging,* 1988.
4. Mancuso AA, Hansberger HR. *Workbook for MRI and CT of the head and neck,* 2nd ed. 1989.
5. Som PM, et al. Chronically obstructed sinonasal secretions: observations on T1 and T2 shortening. *Radiology* 1989;172:515–520.
6. Zinreich SJ, et al. Fungal sinusitis: diagnosis with CT and MR imaging. *Radiology* 1988;169:439–444.

Submitted by: Laura S. Hemann, M.D., and Yutaka Sato, M.D., University of Iowa Hospitals and Clinics, Iowa City, Iowa; Rosalind B. Dietrich, M.B., Ch.B., Senior Editor.

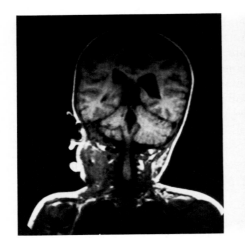

FIG. 54A. SE 516/20.

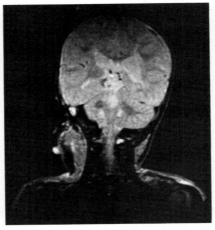

FIG. 54B. SE 2,000/100.

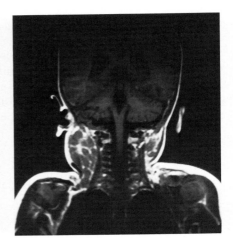

FIG. 54C. SE 583/20 with Gd-DTPA.

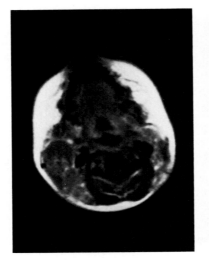

FIG. 54D. SE 583/20 with Gd-DTPA.

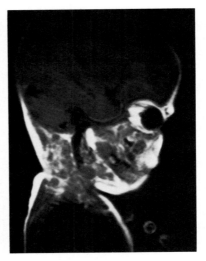

FIG. 54E. SE 450/20 with Gd-DTPA.

Clinical History

A 21-month-old male with a history of histiocytosis X diagnosed 6 months ago that responded well to chemotherapy. At the time of this examination, the patient presented with new, rapidly enlarging bilateral neck masses and fever.

Findings

Figure 54A is a coronal T1-weighted image demonstrating bilateral cervical masses, right greater than left, involving the region of the posterior triangle lymph node chain. These masses are hypointense to fat and slightly hyperintense to muscle. Figure 54B, a T2-weighted coronal image, again demonstrates the bilateral masses, which are hyperintense to muscle and roughly isointense to fat.

Figures 54C–E are T1-weighted post-gadolinium images obtained in coronal, axial, and sagittal planes, respectively. These images again show the bilateral masses with involvement of the posterior triangle, internal jugular, and retropharyngeal lymph node chains. Slight reticular enhancement of the masses is seen following gadolinium administration, and the multicentric nature of the masses is well demonstrated.

Diagnosis

Acute lymphoblastic leukemia with infiltration of cervical lymph nodes.

Discussion

Leukemia is the most common form of childhood cancer, and 97% of cases are acute lymphocytic or acute nonlymphocytic in type. Early manifestations are usually nonspecific, such as anorexia, irritability, and lethargy, and are of short duration at the time of presentation. Progressive failure of normal bone marrow function leads to pallor, bleeding, and fever. Physical examination may reveal lymphadenopathy, splenomegaly or hepatomegaly, and occasionally bone tenderness. When leukemic meningeal involvement is present, headache and vomiting may be seen.

Differential diagnosis includes infectious processes, such as mononucleosis and cat-scratch fever, histiocytosis, and other neoplasms frequently seen in the neck region in children, such as rhabdomyosarcoma.

In our opinion, the primary imaging study for evaluation of cervical lymphadenopathy is contrast-enhanced CT, with MR currently playing an adjunctive role. Lymph nodes are typically isointense to slightly hyperintense to skeletal muscle and much less intense than fat on T1-weighted images. On T2-weighted images, nodes have much higher signal intensity than skeletal muscle and are isointense to slightly hyperintense to fat (1).

References

1. Mancuso AA, Dillon WP. MRI of the head and neck: the neck. *Radiol Clin North Am* 1989; 27:407–420.
2. Som PM. Lymph nodes of the neck. *Radiology* 1987;165:593–600.

Submitted by: Yutaka Sato, M.D., University of Iowa Hospitals and Clinics, Iowa City, Iowa; Rosalind B. Dietrich, M.B., Ch.B., Senior Editor.

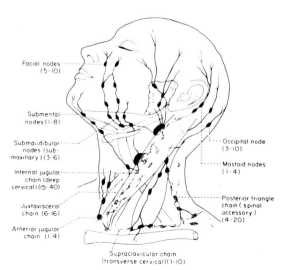

DIAGRAM 1. The palpable cervical lymph node chains with the number of nodes in each chain in parentheses. The deeper chains, including the retropharyngeal and juxtavisceral chains, are not included (2).

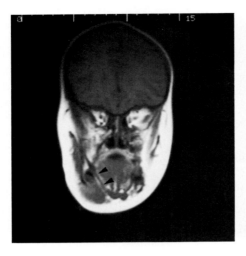

FIG. 55A. SE 383/20.

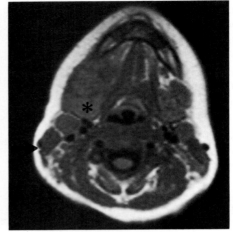

FIG. 55B. SE 383/20.

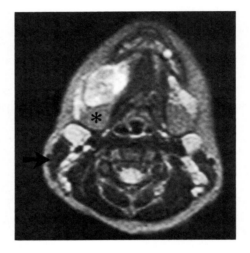

FIG. 55C. SE 2,000/100.

Clinical History

A previously healthy 30-month-old female presented with a 2 × 3 cm firm right submandibular mass, with overlying erythema and induration. A low-grade fever and enlarged tonsils were also noted.

Findings

In the coronal T1 image, a mass is present in the right submandibular space, demarcated laterally by the mandible, superiorly by the mylohyoid muscle (*arrows*), and medially by the anterior digastric muscle belly.

Axial T1- and T2-weighted views of the same area reveal multiple, discrete, well-marginated masses present in the bilateral jugulodigastric and submandibular regions. The largest mass is located anterior to the right submandibular salivary gland (*asterisk*) and measures 4 × 4 × 4.6 cm. Between the sternocleidomastoid muscle (*arrow*) and the submandibular gland are bilateral masses most likely representing enlarged jugulodigastric lymph nodes. The masses are isointense to the masticator muscle on short TR images and inhomogeneously hyperintense to the muscle on long TR images.

The right submandibular gland is displaced posteriorly and medially with normal signal intensity (*asterisk*). The bellies of the anterior digastric muscles are both displaced to the left in the coronal view.

Multiplicity, signal characteristics, and location suggest these masses represent hypertrophied lymph nodes. The inhomogeneity of the largest mass suggests central necrosis.

Incidentally noted are enlarged tonsils that have high signal intensity on T2-weighted images.

The largest mass and the right submandibular gland were surgically resected.

Microscopic analysis revealed a caseating necrotizing granuloma of lymph node with periglandular fibrosis and inflammation of the right submandibular salivary gland. Acid fast and fungi stains, as well as cultures, were negative.

Diagnosis

Probable cat-scratch fever.

Discussion

Three to six lymph nodes form the submandibular group, which drains the lateral chin, lips, cheek, nose, gums, teeth, palate, anterior tongue, and submandibular and sublingual salivary glands (1).

T1 and T2 relaxation times are generally similar for both normal and pathologic nodes. Size is the best criterion to distinguish nodal involvement either by neoplasm or inflammation. However, no definite distinction between malignant and reactive nodes can be made (2). The degree of inflammation, fibrosis, or necrosis present affects the water content of both benign and malignant nodes (3). Both may exhibit necrotic centers that appear as areas of high signal intensity on T2-weighted images (1). In the submandibular group as well as the upper jugular chain nodes, reactive nodes may be fairly large in size.

In general, benign tumors are associated with intact anatomy and tissue planes. In this case, the anterior digastric muscle bellies and the right submandibular salivary gland are displaced without evidence of infiltration.

Differential diagnosis includes inflammation or neoplasm of the right submandibular lymph node. In a young child, inflammation is much more likely. Also, the presence of bilateral regional lymph node enlargement favors inflammation. A more specific diagnosis is not possible with MR. However, in a patient with negative cultures and granulomas and the relevant history, cat-scratch fever is a likely possibility. Cat-scratch fever presents with minimal systemic illness and enlarged lymph nodes in the axilla and neck and is most frequently seen in children (80%) (4).

References

1. Som PM. Lymph nodes of the neck. *Radiology* 1987;165:593–600.
2. Kassel EE, Keller MA, Kucharczyk W. MRI of the floor of the mouth, tongue and orohypopharynx. *Radiol Clin North Am* 1989;27:331–351.
3. Dooms GC, Hricak H, Moseley ME, et al. Characterization of lymphadenopathy by magnetic relaxation times: preliminary results. *Radiology* 1985;155:691–697.
4. Robbins SL, Cotran RS, Kumar V. *Pathologic basis of disease,* 3rd ed. Philadelphia: Saunders, 1984;291.

Submitted by: Teresa M. Simonson, M.D., and Yutaka Sato, M.D., University of Iowa Hospitals and Clinics, Iowa City, Iowa; Rosalind B. Dietrich, M.B., Ch.B., Senior Editor.

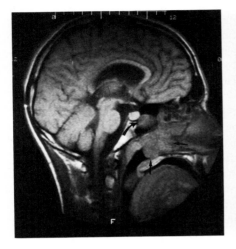

FIG. 56A. SE 450/20.

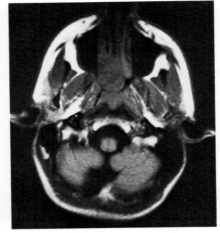

FIG. 56B. SE 516/20.

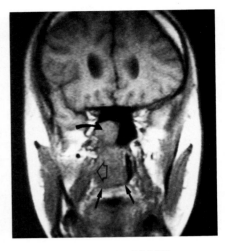

FIG. 56C. SE 383/20.

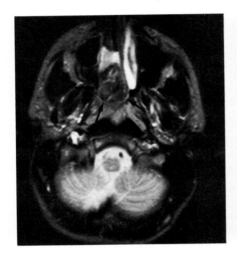

FIG. 56D. SE 2,000/100.

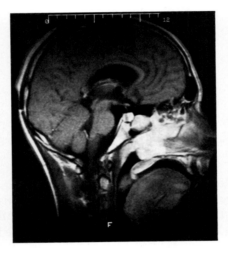

FIG. 56E. SE 450/20 with Gd-DTPA.

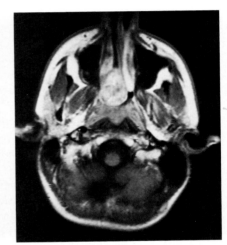

FIG. 56F. SE 516/20 with Gd-DTPA.

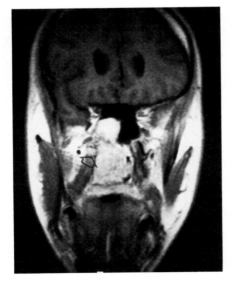

FIG. 56G. SE 383/20 with Gd-DTPA.

Clinical History

A 15-year-old male with 6 months of daily epistaxis and symptoms of nasal obstruction.

Findings

T1-weighted parasagittal (Fig. 56A), axial (Fig. 56B), and coronal (Fig. 56C) images demonstrate a mass that is isointense with adjacent structures within the right posterior nasal cavity and nasopharynx (*arrows*) with sphenoid sinus extension (*curved arrows*). Note the normal-appearing symmetric posterior pharyngeal walls and parapharyngeal space fat on axial view. However, loss of definition along the lateral border of the mass on the coronal scan (*open arrow*) raises a question of extension of the lesion through the palatine bone into the pterygopalatine fossa. Axial T2-weighted MR scan (Fig. 56D) at the level of the upper nasopharynx shows a relatively hypointense, well-circumscribed nasopharyngeal mass (*arrows*) with high signal indicating retained mucus in the right nasal cavity anteriorly. Finally, sagittal (Fig. 56E), axial (Fig. 56F), and coronal (Fig. 56G) T1-weighted images after administration of gadolinium-DTPA confirm the vascular nature of the nasopharyngeal mass and raise the question of pterygopalatine fossa extension anterior to the level of the pterygoid muscles and posterior to the position of the maxillary antrum.

Diagnosis

Juvenile nasopharyngeal angiofibroma (JNA).

Discussion

The differential diagnosis of a nasopharyngeal mass in adolescence includes benign polyp, lymphangioepithelioma, JNA, rhabdomyosarcoma, and esthesioneuroblastoma. Benign polyps are less common in adolescents than children and may either be inflammatory or allergic. Most arise from the nasal cavity or from the maxillary antrum (as in antrochoanal polyp) and extend posteriorly into the nasopharynx. Lymphoepithelioma is a rare lymphoid and fibrous malignant tumor of the nasopharynx that is locally destructive. Rhabdomyosarcoma occurs most frequently in young children, but may occur in adolescents and tends to extend into sinuses and the infratemporal fossa by way of the pterygopalatine fossa. Esthesioneuroblastoma (olfactory neuroblastoma) arises in sensory receptor cells of the olfactory mucosa high in the nasal cavity or in sinuses. It is very rare and exquisitely radiosensitive.

JNA is the most common nasopharyngeal neoplasm in adolescence. It occurs almost exclusively in adolescent boys, presents with epistaxis or nasal obstruction, is highly vascular, and is considered benign although it is extremely locally invasive. Local spread tends to be via natural fissures and foramina, especially through the pterygopalatine fossa and into the sphenoid sinus (two-thirds of cases) as is seen in this case. CT has been the preferred method for staging of JNA, although MR has also proved quite helpful for staging, especially in the evaluation of skull base and intracranial invasion.

An understanding of pterygopalatine fossa anatomy is extremely important in evaluating tumor extension in lesions such as JNA. It is a small triangular space located between the posterior maxillary antral wall and the rounded anterior fused mass of the pterygoid plates. The fossa contains the pterygopalatine (parasympathetic) ganglion and the terminal portion of the internal maxillary artery. *Eight* bony channels leave the pterygopalatine fossa. Tumor gains access from the nasopharynx via the *sphenopalatine foramen* in the vertical portion of the palatine bone (medial wall of the fossa). It can then extend into the middle cranial fossa either anterosuperiorly via the *inferior orbital fissure* (then intracranially via the orbital apex and superior orbital fissure) or posterosuperiorly via the *foramen rotundum* or the *pterygoid (vidian) canal*. Tumor often extends laterally into the infratemporal fossa via the *pterygomaxillary fissure*. Less important routes of spread are anteroinferiorly into the oropharynx by way of the *lesser* and *greater palatine canals* and posteroinferiorly into the nasopharynx via the *palatovaginal (pharyngeal) canal.*

References

1. Osborn AG. The pterygopalatine (sphenomaxillary) fossa. In: Bergeron RT, Osborn AG, Som PM, eds. *Head and neck imaging excluding the brain.* St. Louis: C. V. Mosby, 1984;172–185.
2. Silver JA, Sane P, Hilal SK. CT of the nasopharyngeal region: normal and pathologic anatomy. *Radiol Clin North Am* 1984;22:161–176.
3. Braun IF. MRI of the nasopharynx. *Radiol Clin North Am* 1989;27:315–330.

Submitted by: Martin Crain, M.D., and Yutaka Sato, M.D., University of Iowa Hospitals and Clinics, Iowa City, Iowa; Rosalind B. Dietrich, M.B., Ch.B., Senior Editor.

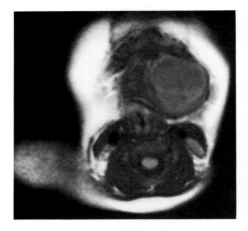
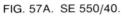

FIG. 57A. SE 550/40.

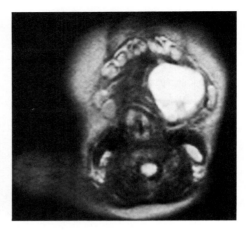

FIG. 57B. SE 1,700/80.

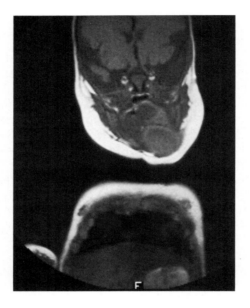

FIG. 57C. SE 683/40.

Clinical History

A previously healthy $2\frac{1}{2}$-month-old white male presented with a sudden onset of high fever and swelling of the left submandibular area. The patient was treated with antibiotics but without response. At admission, the white count was 27,000 with a normal differential.

Findings

A well-demarcated, multilocular cystic mass with some internal debris extends along the left side of the base of the tongue into the submandibular space. It demonstrates intermediate signal on the T1-weighted images (Figs. 57A and C) and high signal on the T2-weighted images (Figs. 57B) and is distinct from the submandibular gland, which is displaced laterally. The mass compresses the vallecula and the upper airway.

Diagnosis

Diving or plunging ranula.

Discussion

Ranula is a benign cystic mass resulting from an obstructed sublingual or minor salivary gland. If it is confined to the sublingual space, it is called a simple ranula. When it extends into the submandibular or parapharyngeal space, it is called a diving or plunging ranula. The distinction is important because surgical therapy requires complete resection. In addition, the distinction of the mass arising from the submandibular space versus that from the sublingual and the floor of the mouth will allow formulation of the appropriate differential diagnosis.

The mylohyoid muscle, which extends from the inferior aspect of the mandible to the hyoid bone, is the landmark that separates the sublingual space and the floor of the mouth superomedially, and the submandibular space inferolaterally. The paired sublingual spaces are on either side of the midline genioglossus muscle. At the posterior margin of the mylohyoid muscle, there are no facial borders limiting the sublingual and submandibular spaces, thus allowing free communication between these spaces. At this same region, these spaces also communicate with the parapharyngeal space as the parapharyngeal space is located posteromedially.

Differential diagnosis includes cystic hygroma, second branchial cleft cyst, thyroglossal duct cyst, inflammatory lesions, and neoplastic lesions, which include dermoid/epidermoid cysts and predominantly necrotic squamous cell carcinoma malignant adenopathy (1).

Cystic hygromas arise from abnormal development of fetal lymphatic tissue. They are usually located in the cervical region (3), which includes the posterior triangle and/or submandibular space, and have no relation to the sublingual space.

Second branchial cleft cysts arise from incomplete obliteration of the embryonic branchial apparatus. They are usually located along the anterior border of the sternocleidomastoid muscle at the level of the mandibular angle. They also have no relation to the sublingual space.

Thyroglossal duct cysts arise from incomplete obliteration of the embryonic thyroglossal duct. They are at anterior midline, usually at the level of the hyoid bone, and embedded in the strap muscle.

Inflammatory lesions, which sometimes can be indistinguishable from malignancy, usually have involvement of multiple spaces and/or of the skin. The presence of calculi on plain film or CT also favors the inflammatory processes (2).

Epidermoid cysts are simple cysts lined by simple epithelial and fibrous tissue. If they are located within the sublingual spaces, they cannot be differentiated radiographically from ranula.

Dermoid cysts are similar to epidermoid cysts but containing various skin elements, thus contributing to different signals on MR.

Squamous carcinoma adenopathy is predominantly of the submandibular group. They tend to have thick irregular walls, compared to thin walls in ranulas. Usually by the time metastatic adenopathy is present, the primary tumor is obvious as the metastatic adenopathy occurs late in oral carcinoma. However, if the primary is not apparent, radiographic distinction between inflammatory lesions and malignant adenopathy may be impossible (1).

References

1. Coit WE, Harnsberger HC, Osborn AG, Smoker WRK, Stevens MH, Lufkin RB. Ranulas and their mimics: CT evaluation. *Radiology* 1987;163:211–216.
2. Kassel EE, Keller MA, Kucharczyk W. MRI of the floor of the mouth, tongue and orohypopharynx. *Radiol Clin North Am* 1989;27:331–351.
3. Silverman PM, Korobkin M, Moore AV. Case report. CT diagnosis of cystic hygroma of the neck. *J Comput Assist Tomogr* 1983;7:519–520.
4. Tabor EK, Curtin HD. MR of the salivary glands. *Radiol Clin North Am* 1989;27:379–392.

Submitted by: Duc Tran, M.D., and Yutaka Sato, M.D., University of Iowa Hospitals and Clinics, Iowa City, Iowa; Rosalind B. Dietrich, M.B., Ch.B., Senior Editor.

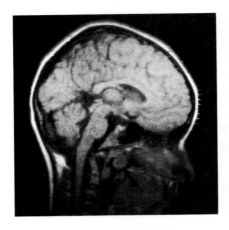

FIG. 58A. SE 550/26.

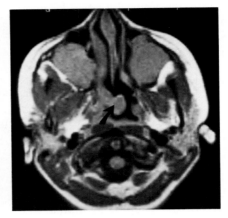

FIG. 58B. SE 933/26.

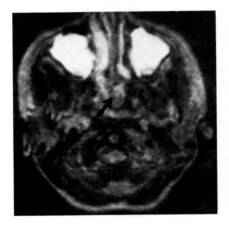

FIG. 58C. SE 2,216/80.

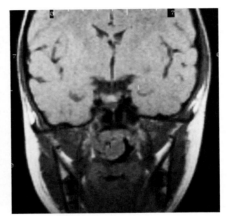

FIG. 58D. SE 1,066/26.

Clinical History

An 11-year-old girl presents with a long-standing history of nasal obstruction, sinus infections, and a right nasopharyngeal mass visualized on physical exam.

Findings

On T1-weighted images a lobulated mass is seen protruding into the nasopharynx (Figs. 58A and D). The mass has low to intermediate signal intensity, higher than that of muscle. The maxillary antra are opacified bilaterally and have intermediate signal intensity (see Fig. 58B). On T2-weighted images, the nasopharyngeal mass is intermediate in signal intensity, having approximately the same signal intensity as subcutaneous fat (see Fig. 58C). The contents of the maxillary antra demonstrate high intensity suggesting retained mucus in the maxillary antra.

Diagnosis

Antrochoanal polyp.

Discussion

Antrochoanal polyp is seen in patients with chronic maxillary antrum disease, often secondary to such processes as chronic sinusitis and allergic diathesis (2). As chronic infection of the maxillary sinuses can be asymptomatic, lack of history of chronic sinusitis in a patient with antrochoanal polyp is not unusual (4). An antrochoanal polyp classically arises from the inflamed edematous mucosa of the lateral wall of the maxillary sinus, although rarely they can also arise from the posterior and superior aspects of the maxillary antrum. The inflamed edematous mucosa develops into an intramural cyst that begins to expand (1). When the intramural cyst has totally occupied the maxillary antrum it herniates through the maxillary ostium into the middle meatus and then into the posterior choana with possible extension into the nasopharynx, where it may hang down into the oropharynx.

Pathologically, the antrochoanal polyp is a large, gray-white, firm, nontender, smooth, bilobed polyp with a long stalk (3).

Commonly, the antrochoanal polyp is unilateral. It accounts for 4%–6% of all nasal polyps in the general population and is found most often in children and young adults, where it accounts for 33% of all nasal polyps. The antrochoanal polyp shows a slight preponderance in males. Classically, a patient's symptoms include nasal obstruction and sometimes rhinorrhea and may be present for a variable length of time before diagnosis. On anterior rhinoscopy a unilateral intranasal polyp is seen that may extend into the nasopharynx (2).

On sinus films, a combination of roentgenographic findings are seen that, taken together, are characteristic of antrochoanal polyps (7). First, antral opacification is identified and usually unilateral, although bilateral antral opacification may also be present. Next, bony expansion without bony erosion of the maxillary antrum is present. Finally, a soft tissue mass is seen within, but not arising from, the nasopharynx.

The definitive surgical treatment for antrochoanal polyp that minimizes recurrence is a Caldwell-Luc approach with concomitant intranasal polypectomy and antrostomy. In patients who undergo intranasal polypectomy by avulsion alone, the antrochoanal polyp often recurs.

Differential diagnosis includes normal or hypertrophied inferior turbinates, chronic hypertrophic polypoid rhinosinusitis, juvenile nasopharyngeal angiofibroma, encephalocele, mucus retention cyst, mucocele, cystic fibrosis, ciliary dysmotility, and malignant tumors of the nasopharynx such as rhabdomyosarcoma (7).

References

1. Berg O, Carenfelt C, Silfversward C, Sobin A. Origin of the choanal polyp. *Arch Otolaryngol Head Neck Surg* 1988;114:1270–1271.
2. Chen JM, Schloss MD, Azouz ME. Antro-choanal polyp: a 10-year retrospective study in the pediatric population with a review of the literature. *J Otolaryngol* 1989;18:168–172.
3. Clegg TJ, Clark WD. Resident's page—pathological quiz case—antrochoanal polyp. *Arch Otolaryngol* 1985;111: 634–636.
4. Crowe JE, Sumner TE, Ramquist NA, Koufman JA. Antrochoanal polyps. *Southern Med J* 1982;75:674–676.
5. Nino-Murcia M, Rao VM, Mikaelian DO, Som P. Acute sinusitis mimicking antrochoanal polyp. *AJNR* 1986; 7:513–516.
6. Shapiro MD, Som PM. MRI of the paranasal sinuses and nasal cavity. *Radiol Clin North Am* 1989;27:447–475.
7. Towbin R, Dunbar JS, Bove K. Antrochoanal polyps. *AJR* 1979;132:27–31.

Submitted by: Michael D'Alessando, M.D., and Yutaka Sato, M.D., University of Iowa Hospitals and Clinics, Iowa City, Iowa; Rosalind B. Dietrich, M.B., Ch.B., Senior Editor.

CASE 59

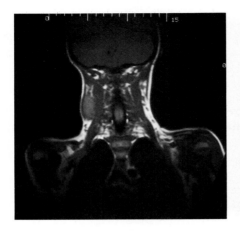

FIG. 59A. SE 450/20.

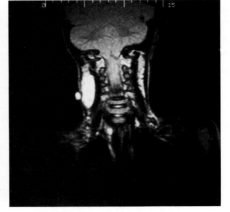

FIG. 59B. SE 2,000/100.

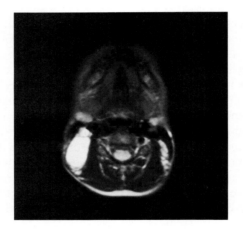

FIG. 59C. SE 2,000/100.

Clinical History

A 33-month-old boy presenting with enlargement of the right side of his neck.

Findings

There is a 3 × 2 cm, multiloculated mass with septations involving the posterior triangle and supraclavicular space. On T1-weighted images, the lesion intensity is greater than that of CSF and muscle, and less than that of fat (Fig. 59A). On T2-weighted images, the mass is bright, with signal intensity greater than that of muscle, fat, and CSF (Fig. 59B). Within the lesion, a fluid-fluid level is visualized (Fig. 59C).

Diagnosis

Cystic hygroma.

Discussion

Cystic hygromas are developmental tumors of lymphatic origin, accounting for 5%–6% of benign tumors in infants and children. Seventy percent occur in the neck, 20% in the axilla, and 5% in other locations such as the mediastinum, retroperitoneum, pelvis, groin, liver, and spleen. Hygromas usually present early, 50%–60% before 1 year of age, 90% before 2 years. They typically present as asymptomatic, fluctuant neck masses. Secondary symptoms may include dysphagia, airway obstruction, infection, or hemorrhage.

On plain films, cystic hygromas are masses of uniform density with round contour and smooth, sharp margins. On ultrasound studies as seen in this case, characteristic MR findings of hygromas are a multiloculated or septated mass, bright on T1-weighted images and very bright on T2-weighted images, usually with a fluid-fluid level with the cyst, caused by the presence of hemoglobin degradation products and increased protein contents secondary to recurrent hemorrhage.

In a differential diagnosis, cystic hygromas need to be differentiated from other cystic masses of the neck. Branchial cleft cysts have a similar MR signal, i.e., relative low intensity on T1-weighted images, high signal intensity on T2-weighted images. However, these are located anterolateral to the carotid sheath, displacing the sternocleidomastoid muscle posterolaterally. Thyroglossal duct cysts are very intense on T2-weighted images, and always located near the midline, along the course of the embryonic thyroid tissue in the anterior neck. Hemangiomas have intermediate T1 signal intensity, bright T2 signal intensity, with surrounding fat, and focal signal void areas due to the presence of vessels or phleboliths. Less likely considerations include abscess, resolving hematoma, salivary gland tumor, thymoma, lymphoma, and teratoma.

References

1. Sheth S, Nussbam S, Hutchins GM, Sanders RC. Cystic hygromas in children: sonographic-pathologic correlation. *Radiology* 1987;162:821–824.
2. Silverman PM, Korobkin M, Moore AV. CT diagnosis of cystic hygromas of the neck. *J Comput Assist Tomogr* 1983;7:519–520.
3. Emery PJ, Bailey CM, Evans JNG. Cystic hygromas of the head and neck. *J Laryngol Otol* 1984;98:613–619.
4. Mancuso AA, Dillon WP. MRI of the head and neck: the neck. *Radiol Clin North Am* 1989;27:407–434.
5. Seigel MJ, Glazer HS, St. Amour TE, Rosenthal DD. Lymphangiomas in children: MR imaging. *Radiology* 1989;170:467–470.

Submitted by: L. Buehner, M.D., and Yutaka Sato, M.D., University of Iowa Hospitals and Clinics, Iowa City, Iowa; Rosalind B. Dietrich, M.B., Ch.B., Senior Editor.

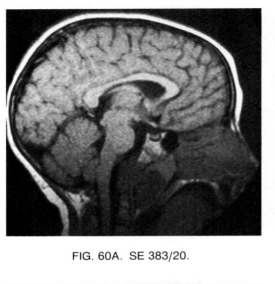

FIG. 60A. SE 383/20.

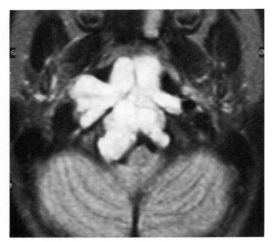

FIG. 60B. SE 2,000/100.

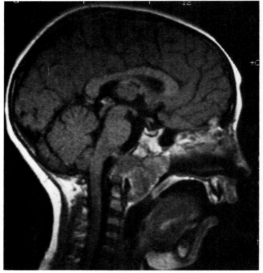

FIG. 60C. SE 383/20 with Gd-DTPA.

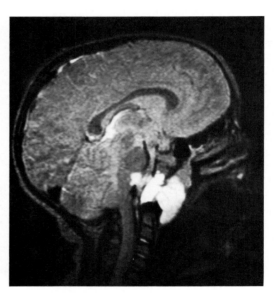

FIG. 60D. SE 2,000/100.

Clinical History

A healthy 5-year-old female with a nasopharyngeal mass discovered on routine physical exam.

Findings

A large mass is present arising from the clivus. It is of low signal on T1-weighted images and demonstrates irregular enhancement following administration of gadolinium-DTPA. On T2-weighted images, it is of homogeneously high signal. The mass extends anteriorly into the nasopharynx and laterally into the petrous apices.

Diagnosis

Clivus chordoma.

Discussion

Chordomas are tumors that arise from the primitive notochord. They are most commonly found in the sacrococcygeal region (50%), but approximately 40% arise in the spheno-occipital region. It is the most common tumor of the clivus. Chordomas may also arise from a vertebral body, most commonly one located in the cervical spine. The peak age for a clivus chordoma is 40 years, with the sacrococcygeal variety presenting 10–12 years later.

The radiographic hallmark of a chordoma is bone destruction associated with a soft tissue mass. Sacrococcygeal chordomas frequently obtain a large size before they are diagnosed owing to the large size of the pelvic cavity into which they extend. They are of moderate to extremely high signal intensity on T2-weighted images owing to the large amount of mucinous contents and isointense or hypointense on T1-weighted images, and demonstrate heterogeneous enhancement following administration of gadolinium-DTPA.

Histologically they are typically composed of cords of physaliphorous cells floating in a sea of gelatinous matrix.

Differential diagnosis of a clivus chordoma includes rhabdomyosarcoma, eosinophilic granuloma, meningioma, metastasis, chondrosarcoma, lymphoma, and granulocytic sarcoma (chloroma).

References

1. Kendall BE. Cranial chordomas. *Br J Radiol* 1977;50:687–698.
2. Schechter MM. Intracranial chordomas. *Neuroradiology* 1974;8:67–82.
3. Sze G. Chordomas: MR imaging. *Radiology* 1988;166:187–191.

Submitted by: Robert A. Garneau, M.D., University of Iowa College of Medicine, and Yutaka Sato, M.D., University of Iowa Hospitals and Clinics, Iowa City, Iowa; Rosalind B. Dietrich, M.B., Ch.B., Senior Editor.

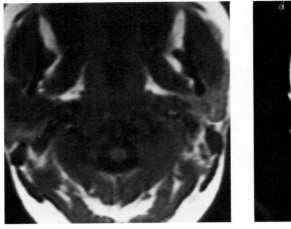 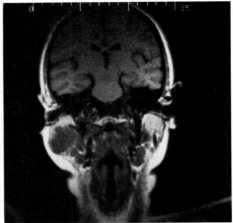

FIG. 61A. SE 416/20.   FIG. 61B. SE 483/20.

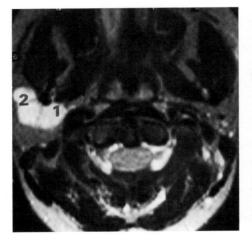 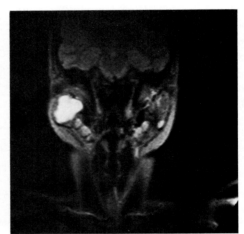

FIG. 61C. SE 2,000/100.   FIG. 61D. SE 2,000/100.

Clinical History

A 16-year-old female with a 2-month history of an enlarging, minimally tender, firm palpable mass overlying the right angle of the mandible. There is no evidence of facial paralysis.

Findings

A 4 × 4 × 3 cm mass extends from the superficial (Fig. 61B) into the deep lobe (Fig. 61A) of the parotid gland but does not involve the parapharyngeal space (PPS).

The mass is relatively homogeneous in appearance with intermediate signal intensity on T1-W (SE 483/20) and high signal intensity on T2-W (SE 2,000/100) images.

Diagnosis

Pleomorphic adenoma (mixed tumor) arising from the superficial portion of the parotid gland.

Discussion

The majority of salivary gland tumors arise in the parotid and are benign in nature. Tumors of the sublingual and submandibular glands occur less frequently and have a higher incidence of malignancy.

Pleomorphic adenomas are the most common benign epithelial tumor of the salivary gland. These tumors are typically asymptomatic and slow growing with a peak incidence in middle age. They tend to be well circumscribed masses with intermediate signal intensity on T1-weighted and high signal intensity on T2-weighted images. Occasionally dystrophic calcification may cause focal areas of signal void within the mass. The presence of calcification, however, more frequently indicates an inflammatory process.

Although evidence of irregular margins, invasion of muscle mass, skull base extension, or enlargement of the facial nerve with nerve paralysis are characteristics strongly supporting malignancy, the majority of carcinomas are well circumscribed and cannot be reliably distinguished from benign neoplasms on the basis of signal characteristics alone.

The course of the facial nerve is used to artificially divide the parotid gland into superficial and deep lobes. The deep lobe insinuates into the fat-filled PPS between the mandibular ramus and styloid process (Diagram 1).

Distinguishing exophytic, deep lobe parotid masses, which extend into the PPS, from a primary PPS tumor is of importance due to the alternative surgical approach, transparotid in the case of the former and transoral in the case of the latter. This distinction may be confidently made if a continuous fat plane is identified separating the deep lobe and mass, indicating extraparotid origin.

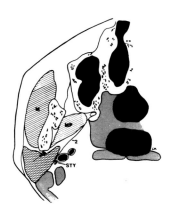

DIAGRAM 1. M = Masseter, MP = Medial Ptergoid, 2 = Parapharyngeal space, Sty = Styloid, Arrow = Facial nerve.

References

1. Tabor ED, Curtin HD. MR of the salivary glands. *Radiol Clin North Am* 1989;27:145–159.
2. Cross RR, Shapiro MD, Som PM. MRI of the parapharyngeal space. *Radiol Clin North Am* 1989;27:353–378.
3. Mandelbluh SM, Braun IF, Davis PC, et al. Parotid masses: MR imaging. *Radiology* 1987;163:411–414.

Submitted by: Michael Hanigan, M.D., and Yutaka Sato, M.D., University of Iowa Hospitals and Clinics, Iowa City, Iowa; Rosalind B. Dietrich, M.B., Ch.B., Senior Editor.

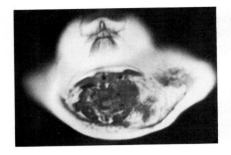

FIG. 62A. SE 1,017/26.

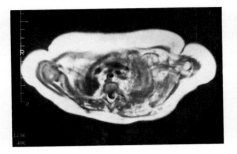

FIG. 62B. SE 1,017/26.

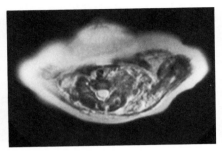

FIG. 62C. SE 2,017/80.

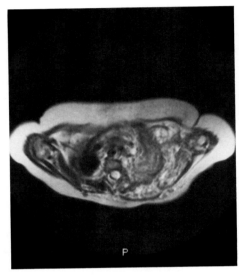

FIG. 62D. SE 2,017/80.

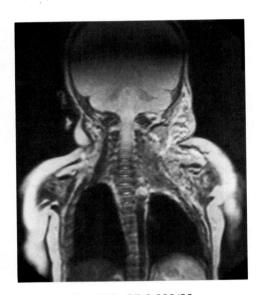

FIG. 62E. SE 2,000/80.

Clinical History

A 1-year-old white female with a history of progressively enlarging soft tissue mass lesion on the left side of the face, neck, and chest.

Findings

Transverse T1-weighted images (Figs. 62A and B) show a very large and poorly defined mass lesion on the left side. The lesion does not appear to be involving the subcutaneous fat of the neck. There is extensive infiltration of muscles with loss of normal tissue planes. The internal structure of the lesion is of mixed low and high signal intensity with a tendency toward a serpiginous appearance.

Transverse (Figs. 62C and D) and coronal (Fig. 62E) T2-weighted images show the extent of this very large lesion. There is varied patchy increase in signal intensity from some areas of the lesion with the T2 weighting. Other areas do not increase in signal intensity.

Diagnosis

Massive hemangioma.

Discussion

Hemangiomas may either be of the capillary or cavernous type. This lesion lacks large vascular lakes characteristic of the cavernous type and is either of the capillary or predominantly capillary type. Some hemangiomas are small and more well defined with a very nonspecific appearance. Several findings in this patient are fairly characteristic of hemangioma and, although not absolutely diagnostic, should suggest the correct diagnosis. These features include the very mottled serpiginous internal structure of the lesion and the varied signal intensity seen on both T1- and T2-weighted pulse sequences. Whereas enlarged feeding and draining vessels may be seen, absence of such vessels does not exclude the diagnosis of hemangioma. The varied internal appearance of this lesion on T1- and T2-weighted images reflects a varied histologic structure. These lesions consist of vascular spaces separated by fibrous stroma. Fat tissue may be present. Areas of calcification may be seen and will have low signal on all pulse sequences. Thrombosis, flowing blood, and hemorrhage with conversion of hemoglobin to hemosiderin all contribute to the marked variation in signal intensity seen within these lesions.

Differential diagnosis includes lymphangitis, fibromatosis, infection, and tumor. Most true tumors of soft tissue have much better defined margins and much more homogeneous internal structure than are seen in this patient. Diffuse infection may have very poorly defined margins as seen in this patient. However, with infection as extensive as in this patient, one would expect to see reactive edema in the adjacent subcutaneous fat, and this is not seen. In addition, infection should have a more uniform low intensity appearance on T1-weighted images with a more uniform pattern on T2-weighted images.

References

1. Sebag GH, et al. Magnetic resonance imaging of pediatric musculoskeletal hemangioma. *AJR* 1989;153:202–207.
2. Cohen JM, et al. Arteriovenous malformations of the extremities: MR imaging. *Radiology* 1986; 156:475–479.
3. Cohen EK, et al. MR imaging of soft tissue hemangiomas: correlation with pathologic findings. *AJR* 1988;150:1079–1081.

Submitted by: Mervyn D. Cohen, M.B., Ch.B., Riley Hospital for Children, Indiana University Medical Center, Indianapolis, Indiana; Rosalind B. Dietrich, M.B., Ch.B., Senior Editor.

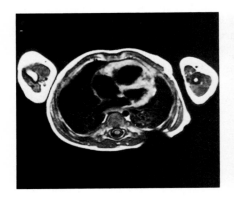
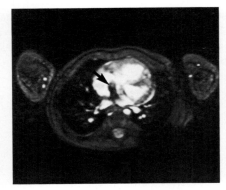
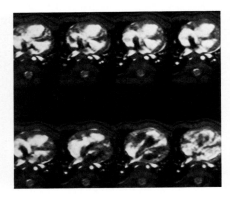

FIG. 63A. SE 500/15.   FIG. 63B. GRE 25/13/30°.   FIG. 63C. SE 25/13.

Clinical History

A 7-month-old infant who was relatively asymptomatic but had a heart murmur. Axial images through the atria (SE 500/15) and a cine study of the atrium were obtained.

Findings

The atrial septum is incomplete. Cine MR images demonstrate a low signal intensity and turbulent jet extending into the right atrium at the site of defect (*arrow*). There is corresponding enlargement of the right ventricle and pulmonary arteries. The left atrium appears normal in size.

Diagnosis

Atrial septal defect.

Discussion

Atrial septal defect is the fifth most common form of congenital heart disease and is one of the most common types of congenital heart disease seen in adults. Most atrial septal defects tend to be large. In most instances, a left-to-right shunt occurs and results in increased volume of blood circulating through the right side of the heart with enlargement of the right atrium, right ventricle, and pulmonary arteries. The right ventricle does not hypertrophy until pulmonary hypertension develops. The atrial pressures are usually equalized. Characteristically, the left atrium is not enlarged as the volume of blood passing through it easily empties back into the right atrium or left ventricle. Patients with large atrial septal defects do not usually develop symptoms early as the left-to-right shunt occurs at low pressure. These shunts are tolerated for decades and are usually picked up as an incident ausculatory finding. The secundum atrial septal defect is the most common type and is located at the junction of the inferior vena cava and right atrium, near the fossa ovalis.

References

1. Diethelm L, Dery R, Lipton MJ, Higgins CB. Atrial-level shunts: sensitivity and specificity of MR in diagnosis. *Radiology* 1987;162:181–186.
2. Lowell DG, Turner DA, Smith SM, et al. The detection of atrial and ventricular septal defects with electrocardiographically synchronized magnetic resonance imaging. *Circulation* 1986;73:89–94.
3. Dinsmore RE, Wismer GL, Guyer D, et al. Magnetic resonance imaging of the interatrial septum and atrial septal defects. *AJR* 1985;145:697–703.

Submitted by: Janet Strife, M.D., Children's Hospital Medical Center, Cincinnati, Ohio; Rosalind B. Dietrich, M.B., Ch.B., Senior Editor.

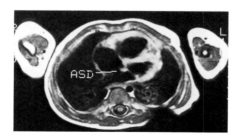

FIG. 63D. SE 500/15.

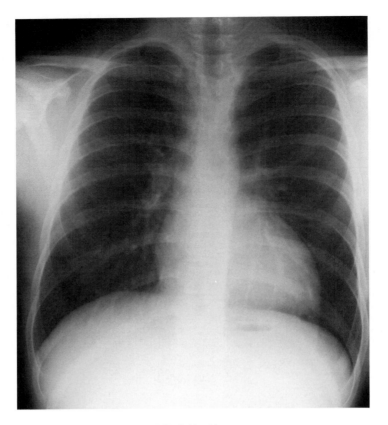

FIG. 64A. X-ray.

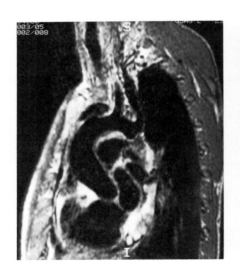

FIG. 64B. SE 800/20.

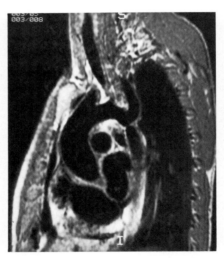

FIG. 64C. SE 800/20.

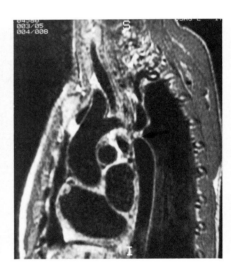

FIG. 64D. SE 800/20.

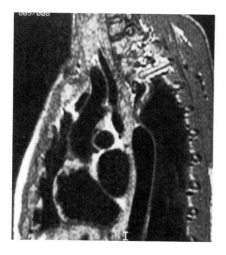

FIG. 64E. SE 800/20.

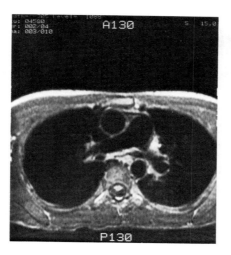

FIG. 64F. SE 800/20.

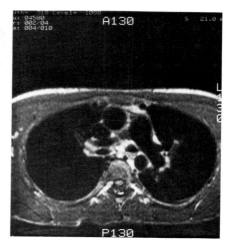

FIG. 64G. SE 800/20.

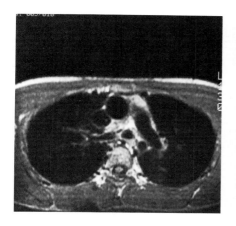

FIG. 64H. SE 800/20.

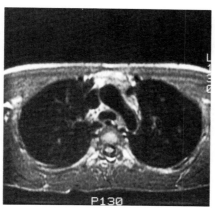

FIG. 64I. SE 800/20.

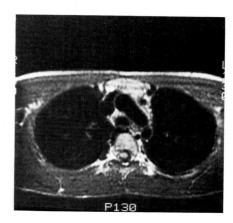

FIG. 64J. SE 800/20.

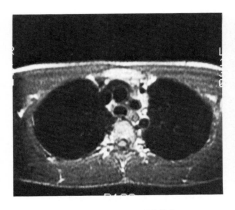

FIG. 64K. SE 800/20.

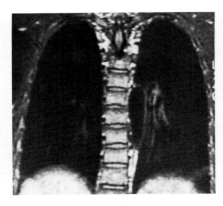

FIG. 64L. SE 769/20.

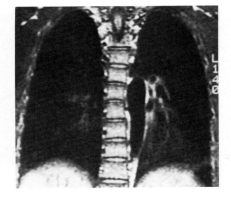

FIG. 64M. SE 769/20.

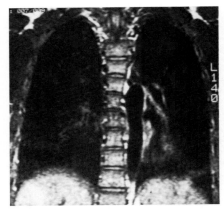

FIG. 64N. SE 769/20.

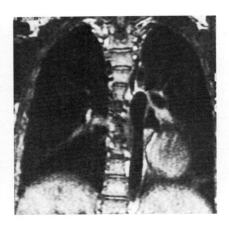

FIG. 64O. SE 769/20.

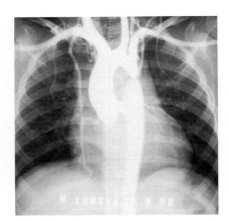

FIG. 64P. X-ray.

Clinical History

A 14-year-old was found to be hypertensive during a routine physical examination.

Findings

Chest x-ray demonstrates that the heart is not enlarged. There is identifiable rib notching on the inferior aspects of the ribs and mild dilatation of the ascending aorta. There is a contour change of the descending aorta with a slight indentation at the site of coarctation with mild post-stenotic dilatation of the descending aorta.

T1-weighted axial, coronal, and sagittal images were obtained. MR anatomy visualized demonstrates a well-defined narrowing of the thoracic aorta distal to the take-off of the left subclavian artery (*arrows*). A discrete indentation or shelf is present that may be asymmetric. Collateral flow to the descending aorta via the intercostal vessels is well demonstrated on the coronal views (*arrowheads*). Dilated internal thoracic arteries can also be seen flowing into the descending aorta. The internal mammary artery is enlarged.

Diagnosis

Coarctation, adult type.

Discussion

Coarctation of the aorta is a congenital anomaly in which there is a narrowing of the aorta that is most commonly located in the region of the ductus arteriosus, at the junction of the aortic arch and descending aorta. In older patients coarctation usually exists as an isolated deficit and is usually postductal in position. When the lesion is a discrete area of narrowing, it is referred to as an adult type coarctation.

Coarctation in infancy is not always an isolated lesion and may be part of more complex anomalies. In infants the narrowing frequently involves a long segment of the aorta in the preductal area or just adjacent to the ductus.

When there is diffuse tubular hypoplasia of the aortic arch and/or aortic atresia, coarctation is referred to as the infantile type.

Other cardiovascular anomalies seen in conjunction with coarctation of the aorta include patent ductus arteriosus and bicuspid aortic valve which is present in 50%–80%. A ventricular septal defect is the most common intracardiac anomaly seen in association with coarctation.

An arteriogram on another patient is included to demonstrate angiographically the discrete coarctation, post-stenotic dilatation, and the collateral flow.

References

1. Baker EJ, Ayton V, Smith MA, et al. Magnetic resonance imaging of coarctation of the aorta in infants: use of a high field strength. *Br Heart J* 1989;62:97–101.
2. Simpson IA, Chung KJ, Glass RF, Sahn DJ, Sherman FS, Hesselink J. Cine magnetic resonance imaging for evaluation of anatomy and flow relations in infants and children with coarctation of the aorta. *Circulation* 1988;78:142–148.
3. von Schulthess GK, Higashino SM, Higgins SS, Didier D, Fisher MR, Higgins CB. Coarctation of the aorta: MR imaging. *Radiology* 1986;158:469–474.

Submitted by: Janet Strife, M.D., Children's Hospital Medical Center, Cincinnati, Ohio; Rosalind B. Dietrich, M.B., Ch.B., Senior Editor.

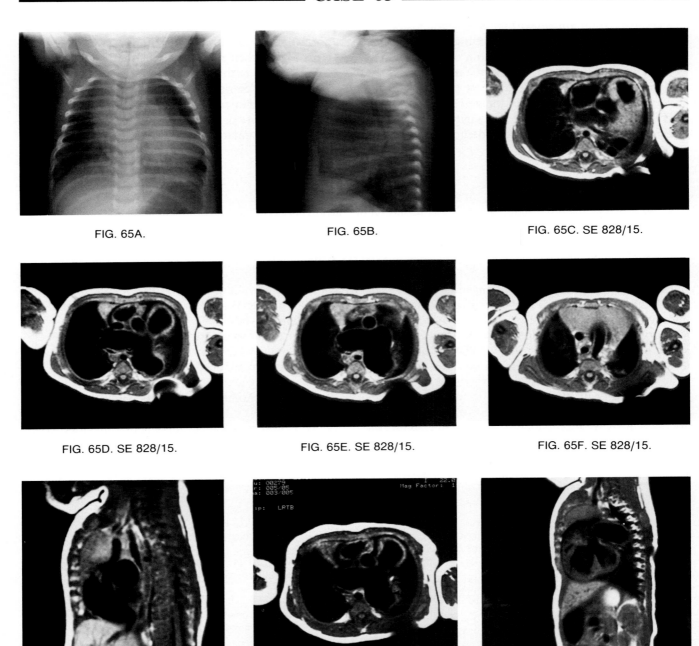

FIG. 65A.

FIG. 65B.

FIG. 65C. SE 828/15.

FIG. 65D. SE 828/15.

FIG. 65E. SE 828/15.

FIG. 65F. SE 828/15.

FIG. 65G. SE 408/15.

FIG. 65H. SE 400/15.

FIG. 65I. SE 408/15.

Clinical History

A term infant with severe respiratory distress and cyanosis.

Findings

The lateral film shows compression of the anterior aspect of the trachea. This is due to marked enlargement of the pulmonary arteries.

Initial sagittal localizing scans were obtained utilizing a SE(408/15) pulse sequence. Subsequently, the same pulse sequence was used to obtain straight axial and axial oblique scans.

A large subaortic ventricular septal defect is noted (*arrow*). There is moderate narrowing in the region of the expected pulmonary valve. However, no definite valve tissue is apparent. The subpulmonic region appears thickened but not obstructed. There is moderate to marked right ventricular hypertrophy. The main, right, and left pulmonary arteries are markedly dilated (*arrowheads*). These are producing compression of both the left and right main stem bronchi (*open arrows*).

Diagnosis

Tetralogy of Fallot variant: absent pulmonary valve with aneurysmal dilatation of the pulmonary arteries.

Discussion

Tetralogy of Fallot with absent pulmonary valve and aneurysmal dilatation of the pulmonary arteries is a distinct entity clinically and radiographically. In 1980 Calder reviewed the literature and found 233 reported cases.

The absent pulmonary valve is associated with moderate to severe pulmonary regurgitation, an obstructed pulmonary valve annulus, subaortic ventricular septal defect, and aneurysmal dilatation of the main and both right and left pulmonary arteries. The pathogenesis of the dilated pulmonary arteries is unknown. The dilated pulmonary arteries may compress the trachea and main bronchi, causing respiratory obstruction. In older patients, the clinical presentation may be one of recurrent respiratory infections and wheezing. Obstructive overdistention of one lung may be seen. The aneurysmal dilatation of the pulmonary arteries may also produce symptoms in the young infant, where the compression involves the anterior aspect of the lower trachea and major bronchi.

Treatment involves early aggressive medical and surgical intervention. Placement of a patient in a semierect prone position or an adjustable tilt table seems to help relieve obstruction. Surgical therapy has included suspension of the pulmonary arteries, resection of the aneurysm, and total repair. Although surgical results in older patients are improving, they have been disappointing in infants.

References

1. Strife JL, Towbin RB, Francis P, et al. Retained fetal lung fluid in two neonates with congenital absence of the pulmonary valve and tetralogy of Fallot. *Radiology* 1981;141:675–677.
2. Arensman FW, Francis PD, Helmsworth JA, et al. Early medical and surgical intervention for tetralogy of Fallot with absence of pulmonic valve. *J Thorac Cardiovasc Surg* 1982;84:430–436.
3. Calder AL, Brandt PW, Barratt-Boyes BG, et al. Variant of tetralogy of Fallot with absent pulmonary valve leaflets and origin of one pulmonary artery from the ascending aorta. *Am J Cardiol* 1980;46:106–116.

Submitted by: Janet Strife, M.D., Children's Hospital Medical Center, Cincinnati, Ohio; Rosalind B. Dietrich, M.B., Ch.B., Senior Editor.

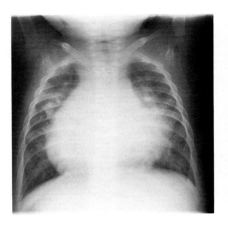

FIG. 66A.

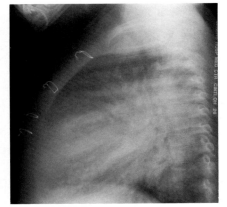

FIG. 66B.

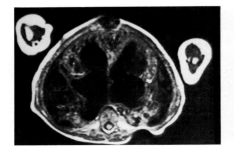

FIG. 66C. SE 545/20.

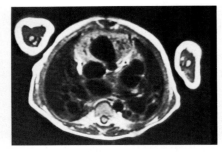

FIG. 66D. SE 545/20.

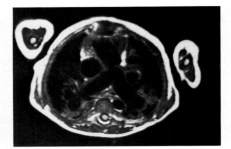

FIG. 66E. SE 545/20.

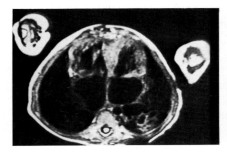

FIG. 66F. SE 545/20.

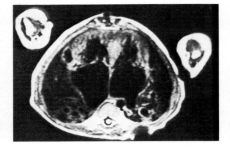

FIG. 66G. SE 545/20.

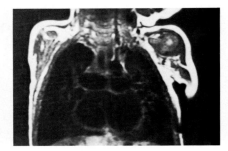

FIG. 66H. SE 545/20.

Clinical History

A 1-year-old white male with congestive heart failure.

Findings

Anteroposterior (AP) and lateral chest radiograph findings: There is gross cardiomegaly with enlargement of right and left atrial chambers. The right atrial enlargement is more evident on the AP film. The left atrial enlargement is demonstrated on the lateral film by posterior displacement of the left main stem bronchus. Additionally, the carina is displayed on the AP film lending further evidence to the presence of left atrial enlargement. There is a bilateral perihilar density consistent with pulmonary edema. Sternotomy wires are in place indicating a previous midline sternotomy. The situs is difficult to evaluate because of the inability to visualize the stomach. The tracheal bifurcation appears to be symmetric, which may indicate situs ambiguous.

Selected axial and coronal T1-weighted, gated scans have been obtained through the heart. The axial scans demonstrate a midline, mesocardiac orientation to the heart. The atrial and ventricular septa are located in a direct AP relationship. The axial image through the pulmonary arteries demonstrates a pulmonary artery band in the mid-portion of the main pulmonary artery (*arrows*) with moderate dilatation of the right and left pulmonary arteries distal to the band. The coronal scans demonstrate a superior atrial septal defect (*open arrow*). The superior vena cava is on the left side (*arrowheads*) and drains into the left-sided atrium. The hepatic veins enter directly into the left-sided atrium from the liver (*curved arrow*). The liver is positioned in the midline. There is bilateral parahilar air-space disease consistent with this patient's diagnosis of pulmonary edema. The pulmonary venous drainage enters the right-sided atrium. Incidental note is made of metallic artifacts in the midline secondary to median sternotomy wires.

Diagnosis

Complex congenital heart disease in association with the asplenia syndrome.

Discussion

In this patient with asplenia, the typical midline liver is identified associated with anomalies of systemic venous and pulmonary venous return. Although this patient has had a previous pulmonary artery banding procedure, the band does not appear to be sufficiently tight to prevent pulmonary edema. MRI may be a useful ancillary imaging technique in mapping out the anatomy prior to attempted surgical intervention in patients with complex congenital heart disease.

Reference

1. Bisset GS III. Cardiovascular system. In: *Magnetic Resonance Imaging in Children.* Cohen MD, Edwards MK, eds. Philadelphia: B. C. Decker, 1990, pp. 541–585.

Submitted by: Janet Strife, M.D., Children's Hospital Medical Center, Cincinnati, Ohio; Rosalind B. Dietrich, M.B., Ch.B., Senior Editor.

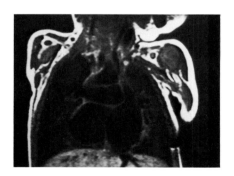

FIG. 66I. SE 545/20.

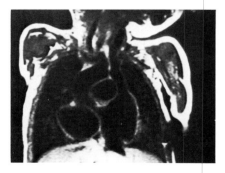

FIG. 66J. SE 545/20.

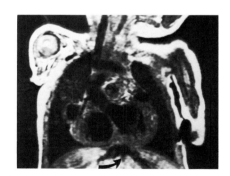

FIG. 66K. SE 545/20.

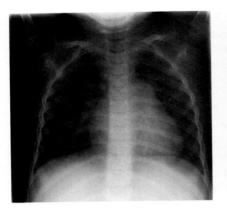

FIG. 67A. X-ray.

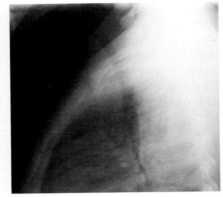

FIG. 67B. X-ray.

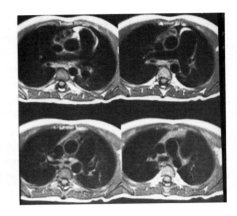

FIG. 67C. SE 652/20.

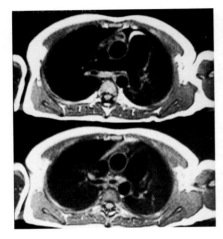

FIG. 67D. SE 652/20.

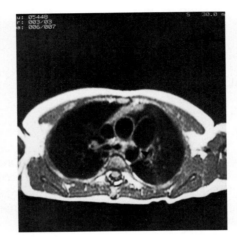

FIG. 67E. SE 652/20.

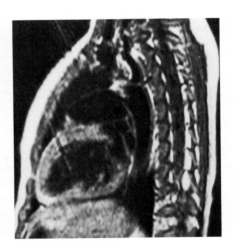

FIG. 67F. SE 652/20.

Clinical History

A 3-year-old white female with a continuous murmur heard throughout systole and diastole. The patient has grown normally.

Findings

On the CXR, the main pulmonary artery appears to be dilated and the left atrium is the upper limit of normal in size. Initial sagittal localizing scans were obtained. Subsequently, axial 5 mm and 3 mm thick sections were obtained through the area of interest below the aortic arch. Coronal and sagittal oblique scans were also obtained through this region. Multiplanar MR images demonstrate moderate dilatation of the main pulmonary artery (*arrows*), the left ventricle, and the left atrium. A ductal diverticulum is seen extending from the proximal descending aorta and is associated with a small patent ductus arteriosus that communicates with the main pulmonary artery (*arrowhead*).

Diagnosis

Patent ductus arteriosus.

Discussion

The ductus arteriosus is a remnant of the distal portion of the left sixth arch and consists of a channel that connects the main pulmonary artery trunk with the descending aorta approximately 5–10 mm distal to the origin of the left subclavian artery. Normal closure of the ductus arteriosus occurs in term infants within the first week of life. In older children, the systemic pressure is higher than the pulmonary artery pressure throughout both systole and diastole. Therefore, left-to-right shunting occurs through a patent ductus arteriosus during both systole and diastole producing a continuous murmur. Patent ductus arteriosus accounts for approximately 10% of all congenital heart disease excluding pre-term infants. Clinical features depend on (a) the size of communication, (b) the relationship between pulmonary and systemic vascular resistance, and (c) the ability of the heart to handle the extra volume. The chest x-ray may demonstrate an enlarged heart and dilated main pulmonary artery together with prominence of the left ventricle and ascending aorta.

In children, treatment usually involves surgical closure of the ductus with division or transection of the ductus since recanalization has been reported following single suture ligation. In preterm infants, the use of indomethacin or other prostaglandin inhibitors to pharmacologically close the ductus has been successful.

Reference

1 Bisset GS III. Cardiovascular system. In: *Magnetic Resonance Imaging of Children.* Cohen MD, Edwards MK, eds. Philadelphia: B. C. Decker, 1990, pp. 541–585.

Submitted by: Janet Strife, M.D., Children's Hospital Medical Center, Cincinnati, Ohio; Rosalind B. Dietrich, M.B., Ch.B., Senior Editor.

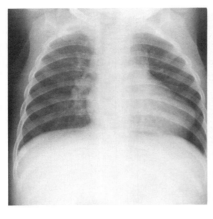

FIG. 68A.

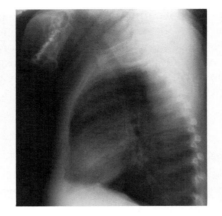

FIG. 68B.

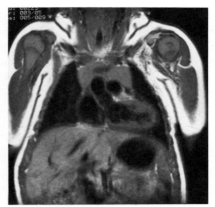

FIG. 68C. SE 889/15.

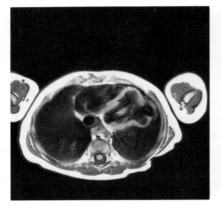

FIG. 68D. SE 889/15.

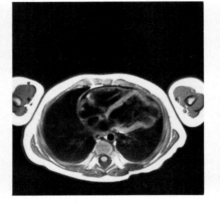

FIG. 68E. SE 889/15.

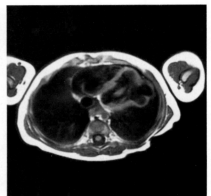

FIG. 68F. SE 889/15.

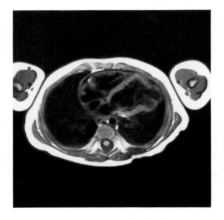

FIG. 68G. SE 889/15.

Clinical History

A 3-month-old female with abnormal pre- and postnatal echocardiograms.

156

Findings

Axial and coronal T1-weighted images were obtained following localizing sagittal scans. A cauliflower-like outpouching is identified at the ventricular apex. The signal within the aneurysm is slightly higher than that coming from the blood in the ventricle, indicating thrombus or very slow flow (which may be difficult to distinguish). The mouth of the outpouching measures slightly more than 2 cm. There is thinning of the ventricular free wall at the same level to approximately 2 mm. The proximal portion of the left coronary artery is identified and appears to be normal.

Diagnosis

Congenital true aneurysm of the left ventricle.

Discussion

Congenital diverticulum or aneurysms of the left ventricle are uncommon. True or false aneurysms can be distinguished as the walls of the latter do not have myocardium within them. The walls of true aneurysms consist of thinned myocardium intermingled with fibrous tissue, whereas those of a false aneurysm are formed only of pericardium. By definition, the wall of a true ventricular diverticulum has all of its layers intact. In practice, this differentiation is difficult as it is based on histopathology, and most of the time, these terms are used interchangeably.

References

1. Freedom RM, Culham JAG, Rowe RD. Diverticulum of a left ventricle. In: Freedom RM, Culham JAG, Rowe RD, eds. *Angiocardiography of congenital heart disease.* New York: Macmillan, 1984;363–367.
2. Singh A, Katkov H, Zavoral JH, Sane SM, McLeod JD. Congenital aneurysms of the left ventricle. *Am Heart J* 1980;99:25–29.
3. Wennevold A, Andersen ED, Efsen F, Jacobsen JR, Lauridsen P. Congenital apical aneurysm of the left ventricle: surgical removal in two infants. *Eur J Cardiol* 1978;7:411–413.

Submitted by: Janet Strife, M.D., Children's Hospital Medical Center, Cincinnati, Ohio; Rosalind B. Dietrich, M.B., Ch.B., Senior Editor.

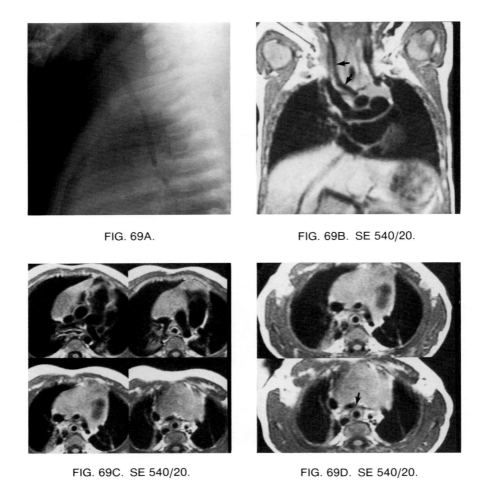

FIG. 69A.

FIG. 69B. SE 540/20.

FIG. 69C. SE 540/20.

FIG. 69D. SE 540/20.

Clinical History

A 4-month-old infant who had recurrent episodes of apnea that occurred with feeding.

Findings

There is focal anterior narrowing of the trachea just at the thoracic inlet. T1-weighted axial, coronal oblique, and axial scans were obtained following initial sagittal localizing scans. Axial images demonstrate a vessel obliquely crossing the anterior aspect of the trachea. The coronal imaging demonstrates that the vessel has its origin in the aortic arch to the left of the midline and crosses the trachea as it ascends into the superior mediastinum (*arrows*). This patient has tracheomalacia secondary to innominate artery compression.

Diagnosis

Innominate artery compression syndrome.

Discussion

Tracheomalacia is a loosely used term that has different meanings for the pediatrician, otolaryngologist, radiologist, and pathologist. It is probably useful to think of tracheomalacia as malfunction of the trachea that may be due to intrinsic or extrinsic causes. Vascular anomalies are one cause of extrinsic compression of the trachea that may lead to intrinsic tracheal stenosis, localized malfunction, and/or both.

The normal innominate artery in children has its origin to the left of the trachea. As it ascends into the mediastinum, it crosses the trachea anteriorly. In a small percentage of children, the innominate artery may cause significant persistent compression of the trachea, causing signs and symptoms of airway obstruction. Stridor, cough, dyspnea, and occasionally cyanosis may occur. Fearon and Shortreed in 1963 coined the term "reflex apnea" to describe episodes of reflex respiratory rest that were noted to occur during feeding in these children.

On lateral films of the neck, there is anterior narrowing of the trachea usually at the level of the thoracic inlet. The mild anterior narrowing of the trachea can be seen in many normal children less than 2 years of age. In symptomatic patients, there is persistent and moderately severe tracheal indentation and collapse. At endoscopy, the tracheal collapse is caused by the pulsating right innominate artery, and frequently abnormal tracheal cartilages are evident.

References

1. Strife JL, Baumel AS, Dunbar JS. Tracheal compression by the innominate artery in infancy and childhood. *Radiology* 1981;139:73–75.
2. Swischuk LE. Anterior tracheal indentation in infancy and early childhood: normal or abnormal? *AJR* 1971;112:12–17.
3. Fearon B, Shortreed R. Tracheobronchial compression by congenital cardiovascular anomalies in children: syndrome of apnea. *Ann Otol Rhinol Laryngol* 1963;72:949–969.
4. Myer C, Auringer ST, Wiatrak B, Bisset GS III. Magnetic resonance imaging in the diagnosis of innominate artery compression of the trachea. *Arch Otolaryngol* (*in press*).
5. Fletcher BD, Dearborn DG, Mulopulos GP. MR imaging in infants with airway obstruction: preliminary observations. *Radiology* 1986;160:245–249.

Submitted by: Janet Strife, M.D., Children's Hospital Medical Center, Cincinnati, Ohio; Rosalind B. Dietrich, M.B., Ch.B., Senior Editor.

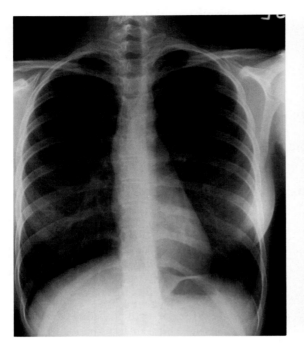

FIG. 70A.

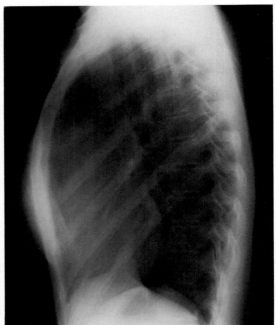

FIG. 70B.

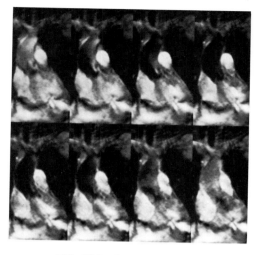

FIG. 70C. GRE 50/13/30°.

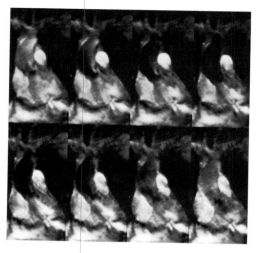

FIG. 70D. GRE 50/13/30°.

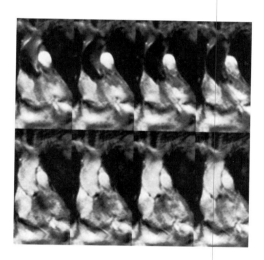

FIG. 70E. GRE 50/13/30°.

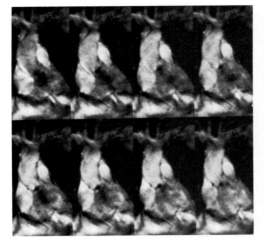

FIG. 70F. GRE 50/13/30°.

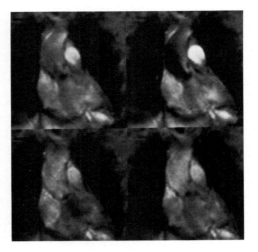

FIG. 70G. GRE 50/13/30°.

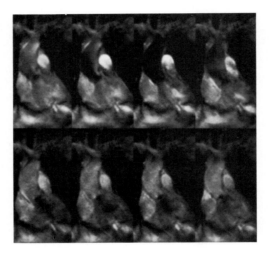

FIG. 70H. GRE 50/13/30°.

Clinical History

The patient was noted to have a cardiac murmur during infancy. She remained asymptomatic until age 5 years when she had two episodes of precordial chest pain associated with exercise. The patient's MR was performed at age 19 years.

Findings

Coronal images were obtained through the plane of the aortic valve. A gradient recalled echo acquisition, (GRE 50/13, 30 degrees), was used. Cine MR demonstrates a turbulent jet of low signal intensity in the ascending aorta during systole. In diastole, a thickened aortic valve is noted as is an aortic regurgitant jet of low signal intensity in the left ventricle. Note the post-stenotic dilatation of the ascending aorta. There is a mild prominence of the ascending aorta seen on posteroanterior film. On the lateral film, there is left ventricular enlargement, as noted by the presence of a left ventricle posterior to the inferior vena cava.

Diagnosis

Aortic stenosis with aortic insufficiency.

Discussion

This patient has congenital mild aortic stenosis and aortic regurgitation. Aortic valvar stenosis accounts for 6% of congenital heart disease in children and can exist as an isolated lesion. Frequently, the aortic valve is bicuspid and aortic leaflets are fused or there is commissural fusion. Left ventricular outflow tract obstruction leads to turbulence, and frequently there is a jet with post-stenotic dilatation of the ascending aorta. In patients with significant aortic insufficiency, there is dilatation of the ascending aorta due to volume load of the regurgitant fraction plus normal left ventricular output. The effect of left ventricular outflow tract obstruction is an increase in left ventricular systolic pressure that is further compounded by the aortic insufficiency. Left ventricular myocardial oxygen requirements are increased and left ventricular fibrosis with subsequent left ventricular dilatation and ultimately congestive heart failure may develop.

Reference

1. Bisset GS III. Cardiovascular system. In: *Magnetic Resonance Imaging of Children.* Cohen MD, Edwards MK, eds. Philadelphia: B. C. Decker, 1990, pp. 541–585.

Submitted by: Janet Strife, M.D., Children's Hospital Medical Center, Cincinnati, Ohio; Rosalind B. Dietrich, M.B., Ch.B., Senior Editor.

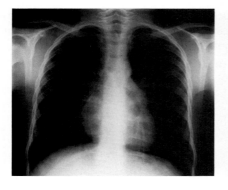

FIG. 71A.

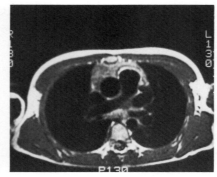

FIG. 71B. SE 667/20.

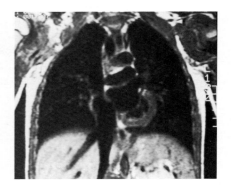

FIG. 71C. SE 667/20.

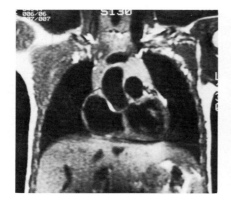

FIG. 71D. SE 667/20.

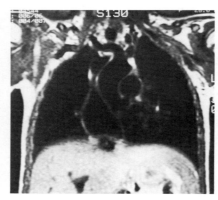

FIG. 71E. SE 667/20.

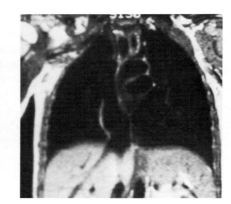

FIG. 71F. SE 667/20.

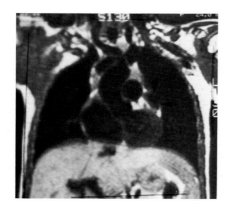

FIG. 71G. SE 667/20.

Clinical History

A 6-year-old patient who had intermittent left pericardial chest pain.

Findings

Following T1-weighted sagittal localizing images, T1-weighted axial and coronal images were obtained. The heart and all of its chambers appear normal in size. The left ventricular myocardium is of normal thickness. The apex of the left ventricle lies within the left costophrenic sulcus. There is prominence of the main pulmonary artery segment. Partial absence of the left pericardium is apparent and the left atrial appendage partially herniates through this defect (*arrows*) and creates the density seen inferior to the pulmonary artery segment, which correlates nicely with plain films.

Diagnosis

Partial absence of the pericardium.

Discussion

Congenital absence of the pericardium may be partial or complete. The pericardial defect represents defective formation of the pleuropericardial membrane, positioned along the lateral heart border, or, if juxtadiaphragmatic, defective formation of the septum transversum.

The chest x-ray is often highly suggestive of the diagnosis. The heart is slightly levoposed, and the left upper border shows three unusual prominent convexities: the aortic knob, main pulmonary artery, and left atrium. The prominent bulge inferior to the pulmonary artery is produced by the herniating left atrial appendage.

The partial forms of pericardial defect may require surgery because there is a risk of herniation and strangulation of the ventricles or left atrial appendage. This diagnosis can be made by MRI.

Complete absence of the pericardium may be associated with underlying congenital heart disease and/or with more severe anomalies such as diaphragmatic defects. Diaphragmatic pericardial defects may be seen in association with a diaphragmatic defect resulting in herniation of the greater omentum or other intraabdominal structures into the pericardial cavity.

References

1. Schiavone WA, O'Donnell JK. Congenital absence of the left portion of parietal pericardium demonstrated by nuclear magnetic resonance imaging. *Am J Cardiol* 1985;55:1439–1440.
2. Rowland TW, Twible EA, Norwood WI Jr, Keane JF. Partial absence of the left pericardium: diagnosis by two-dimensional echocardiography. *Am J Dis Child* 1982;136:628–630.
3. Baim RS, MacDonald IL, Wise DJ, Lenkei SC. Computed tomography of absent left pericardium. *Radiology* 1980;135:127–128.

Submitted by: Janet Strife, M.D., Children's Hospital Medical Center, Cincinnati, Ohio; Rosalind B. Dietrich, M.B., Ch.B., Senior Editor.

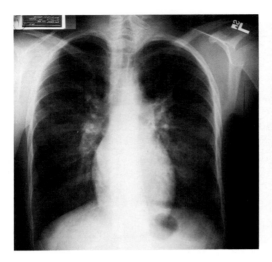

FIG. 72A.

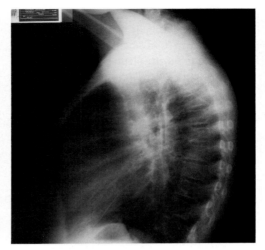

FIG. 72B.

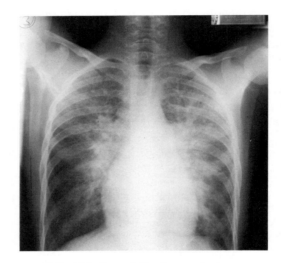

FIG. 72C. X-ray following angiogram.

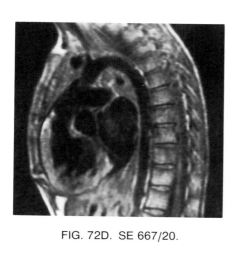

FIG. 72D. SE 667/20.

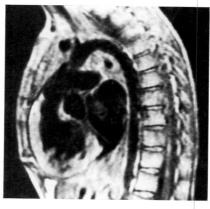

FIG. 72E. SE 667/20.

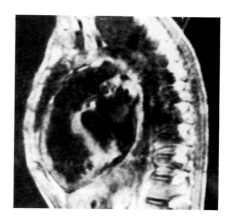

FIG. 72F. SE 667/20.

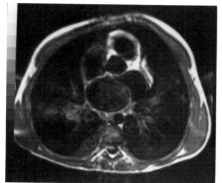

FIG. 72G. SE 667/20.

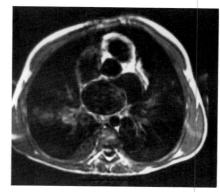

FIG. 72H. SE 667/20.

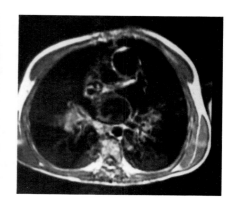

FIG. 72I. SE 667/20.

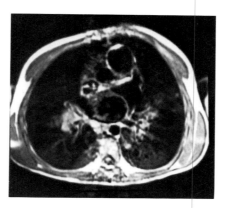

FIG. 72J. SE 667/20.

Clinical History

A 15-year-old patient who was followed for many years with a history of "asthma" associated with moderate exertional dyspnea. The patient had intermittent episodes of hemoptysis.

Findings

The transverse cardiac size is normal on posteroanterior view, but on lateral film, there is right ventricular enlargement. The pulmonary arteries are prominent bilaterally suggesting pulmonary hypertension.

The patient had a cardiac catheterization and the pulmonary artery pressure wedge was 30 mm, with a pulmonary artery pressure of 144/78 mm. Because of severe pulmonary hypertension, only a small amount of nonionic contrast was injected in an attempt to evaluate the pulmonary veins and left atrium. Despite the nonionic injection, the patient developed florid pulmonary edema following this angiogram (Fig. 72C).

Axial and sagittal images 5 mm thick were obtained using a cardiac-gated, spin-echo, multislice technique (TR/TE 667/20).

An accessory chamber was identified posterior to the normal left atrium. Intermediate signal intensity within this chamber indicated slow (obstructive) flow. The pulmonary veins were dilated and emptied into the posterior chamber. Increased signal intensity in the lung parenchyma was most consistent with pulmonary edema. No atrial septal defect was identified.

Diagnosis

At surgery, cor triatriatum was confirmed and an uneventful surgical resection of the fibromuscular diaphragm was performed.

Discussion

Cor triatriatum is a congenital anomaly in which the pulmonary veins are partially obstructed. The obstructing membrane is usually quite thin and can be difficult to image. With marked left atrial pressure increase, there is pulmonary venous pressure increase and pulmonary hypertension may result.

There is usually a single ostium of varying size connecting the chambers. This lesion usually occurs as an isolated malformation, although in approximately one-quarter of cases it is associated with complex congenital heart disease. The pulmonary veins enter the accessory chamber posterosuperiorly with subsequent connection with the true left atrium, atrial appendage, and mitral valve. The accessory chamber may receive only part of the pulmonary venous return and connect with the left atrium through a stenotic ostium. The remaining veins may join the true left atrium.

Clinically, these patients may present in infancy with bronchiolitis and signs of recurrent wheezing. Older children may present with signs of pulmonary hypertension or chronic airway disease.

MRI is effective in delineating the intraatrial membrane. The obstructed flow in the accessory chamber of cor triatriatum was suggested on the basis of increased signal caused by the slow flow.

The differential diagnosis of obstructing pulmonary venous hypertension includes mitral stenosis, left atrial tumors, and pulmonary venous stenosis. MRI may be useful in evaluation of children with unexplained pulmonary hypertension.

References

1. Bisset GS III, Kirks DR, Strife JL, Schwartz DC. Cor triatriatum: diagnosis by MR imaging. *AJR* 1987;149:567–568.
2. Grondin C, Leonard AS, Anderson RC, Amplatz KA, Edwards JE, Varco RL. Cor triatriatum: a diagnostic surgical enigma. *J Thorac Cardiovasc Surg* 1964;48:527.
3. Freedom RM, Culham JAG, Rowe RD. Anomalies of pulmonary venous connections and obstruction to pulmonary venous flow. In: Freedom RM, Culham JAG, Rowe RD, eds. *Angiocardiography of congenital heart disease.* New York: Macmillan, 1984;289–293.
4. Jacobstein MD, Hirschfeld SS. Concealed left atrial membrane: pitfalls in the diagnosis of cor triatriatum and supravalve mitral ring. *Am J Cardiol* 1982;49:780–786.
5. Marin-Garcia J, Tandon R, Lucas RV, Edwards JE. Cor triatriatum: study of 20 cases. *Am J Cardiol* 1975;35:59–66.
6. Lang D, Wagenvoort CA, Kupferschmid C, Kleihauer E. Cor triatriatum masked by primary pulmonary hypertension. *Pediatr Cardiol* 1985;6:161–164.

Submitted by: Janet Strife, M.D., Children's Hospital Medical Center, Cincinnati, Ohio; Rosalind B. Dietrich, M.B., Ch.B., Senior Editor.

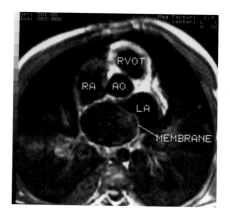

FIG. 72K. SE 667/20.

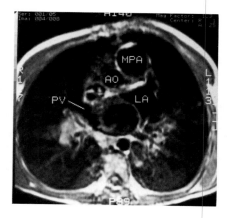

FIG. 72L. SE 667/20.

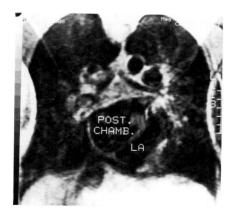

FIG. 72M. SE 667/20.

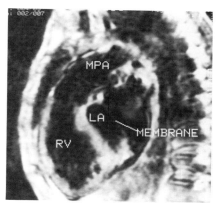

FIG. 72N. SE 667/20.

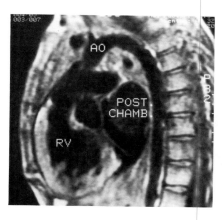

FIG. 72O. SE 667/20.

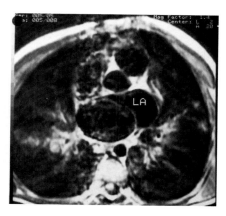

FIG. 72P. SE 667/20.

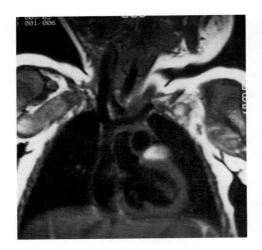

FIG. 73A. SE 500/20.

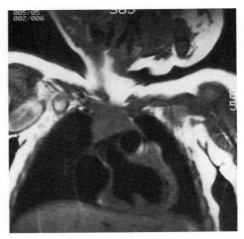

FIG. 73B. SE 500/20.

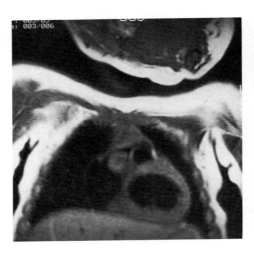

FIG. 73C. SE 500/20.

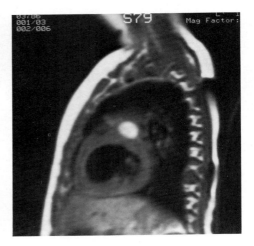

FIG. 73D. SE 462/20.

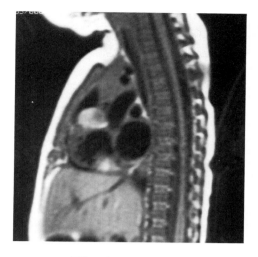

FIG. 73E. SE 462/20.

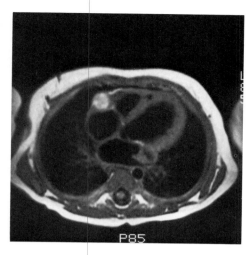

FIG. 73F. SE 500/20.

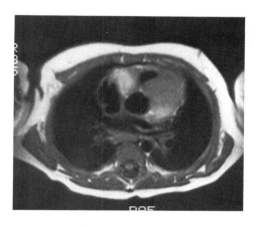

FIG. 73G. SE 500/20.

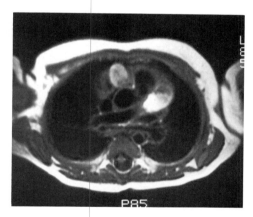

FIG. 73H. SE 500/20.

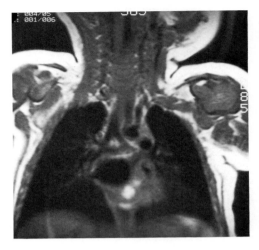

FIG. 73I. SE 500/20.

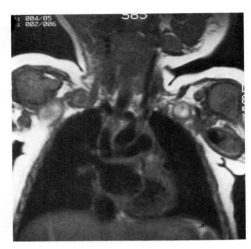

FIG. 73J. SE 500/20.

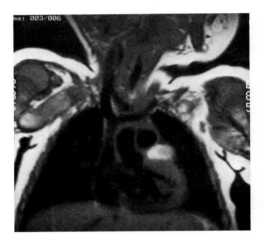

FIG. 73K. SE 500/20.

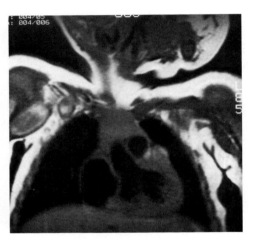

FIG. 73L. SE 500/20.

Clinical History

A patient presented at 3 months of age with tachypnea. The patient had a previous history of fever, lymphadenopathy, and rash.

Initial sagittal localizing scans were obtained utilizing a T1-weighted sequence. Subsequently, axial and coronal scans were also obtained.

Findings

The coronary arteries are diffusely enlarged and contain multiple areas of intermittent signal intensity, which may represent thrombus or markedly slow flow. The largest aneurysm appears to arise from the proximal left coronary artery and measures approximately 1.9 cm in maximal dimension. In addition to the aneurysms evident, there are several fusiform aneurysms present elsewhere in the body. There is involvement of both axillary arteries with large fusiform aneurysms. MR was used to sequentially follow this patient.

A selective right coronary artery injection was performed 4 months prior to the MR scan. Coronary angiography demonstrated the large fusiform aneurysms. The major morbidity and mortality in Kawasaki disease relate to coronary artery aneurysms. Noticing the abnormal flow characteristics in this vessel, one can understand ventricular irritability and/or fatal arrhythmias. These patients may also have myocardial infarcts.

Diagnosis

Kawasaki disease.

Discussion

Kawasaki disease is a multisystem inflammatory disease that characteristically affects infants and young children. Its major associated abnormality is the formation of coronary artery aneurysms, which may be focal or diffuse. Although evaluation of these aneurysms has been based on two-dimensional echocardiography, problems may occasionally arise in using this technique. MR can be used to evaluate the coronary artery aneurysms in patients in whom echocardiography is not technically feasible (small acoustic window or not diagnostic) as in some distal aneurysms. Additional information may be utilized concerning flow characteristics within the coronary artery aneurysms, global extent of other

thoracic aneurysms, and degree of pericardial and/or pleural involvement.

Kawasaki disease was initially described in 1967, and since that time there has been a marked increase in incidence of the disease. The major complication leading to morbidity and mortality is the presence of coronary artery aneurysms, occurring in approximately 10%–20% of patients with this disease.

Flow characteristics within the aneurysmally dilated vessels may be discerned with this technique. In this patient, MRI initially confirmed the presence of angiographically identified slow coronary blood flow. On the later MR evaluation, coronary thrombi were identified.

References

1. Bisset GS III, Strife JL, McCloskey J. MR imaging of coronary artery aneurysms in a child with Kawasaki disease. *AJR* 1989;152:805–807.
2. Kawasaki T. Mucocutaneous lymph node syndrome—clinical observation of 50 cases. *Jpn J Allergy* 1967;16:178–182.
3. Bell DM, Morens DM, Holman RC, Hurwitz MD, Hunter MK. Kawasaki syndrome in the United States. *Am J Dis Child* 1983;137:211–214.
4. Kawasaki T, Kosaki F, Okawa S, Shigematsu I, Yanagawa H. A new infantile acute febrile mucocutaneous lymph node syndrome (MLNS) prevailing in Japan. *Pediatrics* 1974;54:271–276.
5. Rauch AM. Kawasaki syndrome: issues in etiology and treatment. *Adv Pediatr Infect Dis* 1989;4:163–182.
6. Kato H, Inoue O, Akagi T. Kawasaki disease: cardiac problems and management. *Pediatr Rev* 1988;9:209–217.
7. Benson LN, Rowe RD. Predictors of coronary risk in Kawasaki disease. *Prog Clin Biol Res* 1987;250:299–304.

Submitted by: Janet Strife, M.D., Children's Hospital Medical Center, Cincinnati, Ohio; Rosalind B. Dietrich, M.B., Ch.B., Senior Editor.

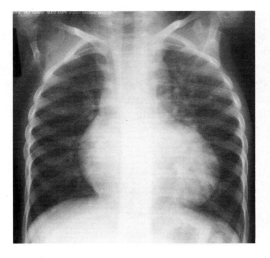

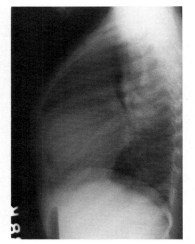

FIG. 74A.

FIG. 74B.

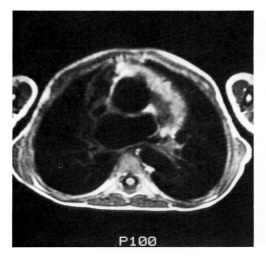

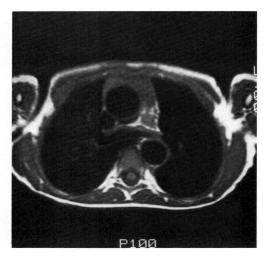

FIG. 74C. SE 545/20.

FIG. 74D. SE 545/20.

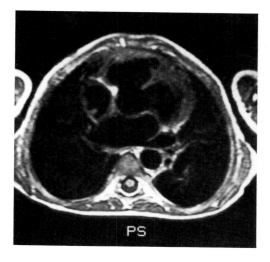

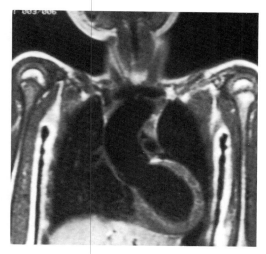

FIG. 74E. SE 545/20.

FIG. 74F. SE 545/20.

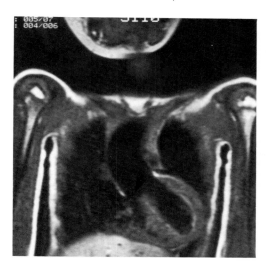

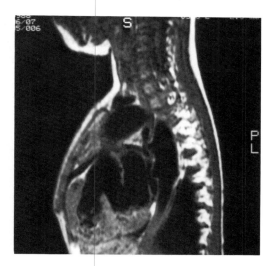

FIG. 74G. SE 545/20.

FIG. 74H. SE 545/20.

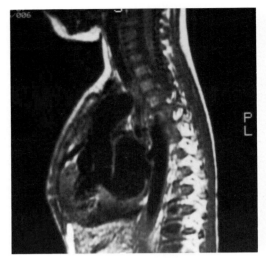

FIG. 74I. SE 545/20.

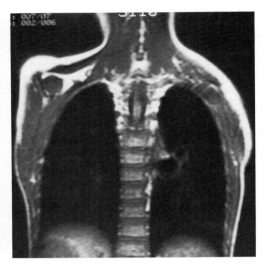

FIG. 74J. SE 545/20.

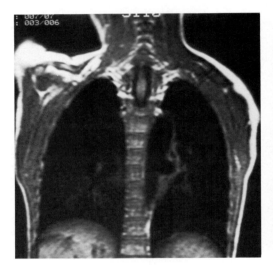

FIG. 74K. SE 545/20.

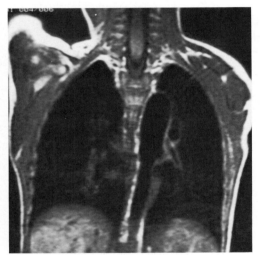

FIG. 74L. SE 545/20.

Clinical History

A 4-year-old patient with cyanosis since birth.

Findings

The plain film demonstrates mild cardiac enlargement. There is a concave segment of the main pulmonary artery. Systemic collateral vessels can be recognized on the basis of the plain film. Particularly, the vessel in the left lower lobe looks larger distally and does not have its origin from the left hilum.

Serial, axial, coronal, parasagittal, and oblique parasagittal images were obtained through the cardiac base. Cardiac-gated T1-weighted images were acquired (TR/TE 545/20). There is no discernible main pulmonary artery or left-to-right pulmonary arteries. The left atrium and left ventricle are enlarged and a subaortic ventricular septal defect is seen. The aorta is also noted to be overriding in its position relative to the interventricular septum (*arrows*). The ascending, transverse, and immediate descending aorta are enlarged compatible with the high flow state consistent with the setting of pulmonary atresia with bronchial collaterals. Large left and right bronchial arterial collaterals arise from the proximal descending thoracic aorta. The aortic caliber just distal to the take-off of these large bronchial collaterals diminishes by approximately 50%. There is nonconfluence of the bronchial vessels from the left lung to the right.

Diagnosis

Severe tetralogy of Fallot: pulmonary atresia, ventricular septic defect (VSD) with systemic collaterals.

Discussion

Pulmonary atresia is present when there is no forward flow through the pulmonic valve. This represents the extreme form of obstruction of the valve and is frequently associated with infundibular stenosis. Nomenclature for this lesion when an associated VSD is present includes such terms as severe tetralogy of Fallot with pulmonary atresia, truncus arteriosus type IV, pseudotruncus arteriosus, and pulmonary atresia with VSD.

Regardless of the terminology, all of these lesions share the common features of discontinuity between the right ventricle and pulmonary arteries. In most of these patients, there are a fibrous remnant between the right ventricle and pulmonary artery and atresia of the valve or an atretic infundibulum. How does blood flow to the lungs? The purpose of imaging in these patients is to characterize the pulmonary blood flow. One needs to determine the presence or absence of the main pulmonary artery and branch pulmonary arteries and whether they are confluent (connected) or not. The sites of origins of the pulmonary arteries need to be identified and the number of collateral vessels evaluated. The presence of a patent ductus arteriosus and its site of origin also have significance. The peripheral pulmonary arteries and proximal main pulmonary artery have separate embryologic derivation. Therefore, it is possible to have a normal pulmonary plexus develop despite discontinuity of the heart and main pulmonary artery.

There is also disagreement with regard to naming the collaterals. They have been termed both bronchial arteries and aortic pulmonary collateral vessels. The collateral flow to the lung may also include large vessels of brachiocephalic origin.

MR is useful in assessing both the extent of collateral flow and the site of origin of the vessels. In order to perform a total repair in a patient with pulmonary atresia and VSD, a main pulmonary artery or large pulmonary artery must be present that can be grafted to the right ventricle. Therefore, the finding of nonconfluent pulmonary vessels is extremely important.

Hemodynamically, these patients have systemic pressure of the right ventricle. Blood flows from the right atrium into the right ventricle and then into the overriding ascending aorta. Subsequently, blood flow via the aortic pulmonary collaterals into the lungs where oxygenation occurs. Blood is then returned to the left atrium with subsequent filling of the left ventricle and then the ascending aorta. The ascending aorta is strikingly enlarged because it has both the systemic and pulmonary venous return entering it.

References

1. Canter CE, Gutierrez FR, Mirowitz SA, Martin TC, Hartmann AF Jr. Evaluation of pulmonary arterial morphology in cyanotic congenital heart disease by magnetic resonance imaging. *Am Heart J* 1989;118:347–354.
2. Mirowitz SA, Gutierrez FR, Canter CE, Vannier MW. Tetralogy of Fallot: MR findings. *Radiology* 1989;171:207–212.
3. Rees RS, Somerville J, Underwood SR, et al. Magnetic resonance imaging of the pulmonary arteries and their systemic connections in pulmonary atresia: comparison with angiographic and surgical findings. *Br Heart J* 1987;58:621–626.

Submitted by: Janet Strife, M.D., Children's Hospital Medical Center, Cincinnati, Ohio; Rosalind B. Dietrich, M.B., Ch.B., Senior Editor.

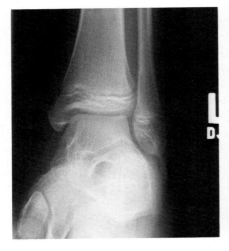

FIG. 75A.

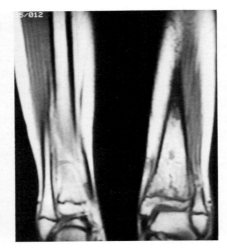

FIG. 75B. SE 300/15.

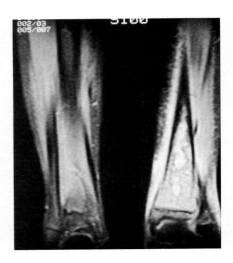

FIG. 75C. IR 1,500/150/20.

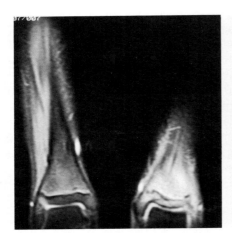

FIG. 75D. IR 1,500/150/20.

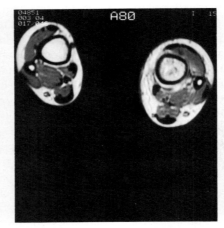

FIG. 75E. SE 2,500/20.

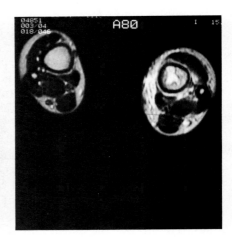

FIG. 75F. SE 2,500/80.

Clinical History

A 12-year-old girl with a 2-week history of pain in the left ankle. History of a bicycle accident 1 week prior to onset of pain.

Findings

Radiograph of the left ankle shows subtle erosion of cortical bone in the medial metaphysis (Fig. 75A).

Coronal MR image (SE 300/15) of the ankles reveals focal low signal intensity in the left metaphysis and epiphysis (Fig. 75B). The physis, which should be seen as a low signal intensity line separating metaphysis and epiphysis, shows some intermediate signal intensity, suggesting that the process in the metaphysis has extended through the physis into the epiphysis.

Coronal short T1 inversion recovery (STIR) image (IR 1,500/150/20) of the left ankle at a similar level shows diffuse increased signal intensity metaphyseal marrow with focal regions of even brighter signal intensity (Fig. 75C). Cortical destruction can be appreciated in the medial mid-metaphyseal region.

Coronal STIR (IR 1,500/150/20) image of the normal right ankle (Fig. 75D). The STIR sequence allows suppression of signal from the fatty marrow. The diffuse increased marrow signal intensity in the distal left tibial metaphysis can be appreciated by comparing the marrow signal of Fig. 75C and D. These findings suggest a diffuse inflammatory process of the left tibial metaphysis with focal areas of either more intense inflammation or fluid.

Axial intermediate-weighted (SE 2,500/20) image through the distal tibias shows marrow heterogeneity in the left tibial metaphysis and strands of decreased signal intensity in the medial subcutaneous fat (Fig. 75E).

Axial T2-W (SE 2,500/80) image at the same level reveals focal increased signal intensity surrounded by a low signal intensity rim that abuts the anterior cortex of the left tibial metaphysis (Fig. 75F). Linear intermediate signal intensity is seen surrounding the anterior and medial cortex of the left tibial metaphysis. This is consistent with cellular periosteal reaction or edema.

Diagnosis

Staphylococcal osteomyelitis of the left tibial metaphysis and epiphysis.

Discussion

Early diagnosis of osteomyelitis is essential in preventing the complications of delayed or inadequate treatment. Risk factors include systemic disease, immunosuppression, and traumatic injury. Osteomyelitis in children typically occurs in the metaphysis, and approximately 80%–85% of cases are caused by staphylococci. *Pseudomonas* can be seen in penetrating injuries and *Salmonella* is common in patients with sickle cell disease.

On MR images, acute osteomyelitis is seen as decreased signal intensity on T1-weighted images, and normal or increased signal intensity on T2-weighted images (1, 2). On T2-weighted images, the abnormality can have an ill-defined interface with normal marrow, or, in approximately one-third of cases, there can be a low signal intensity rim reflecting sclerosis around the focus of infection. Both of these findings can be appreciated in this case. In this patient, the linear increased signal intensity surrounding the cortical bone on the transverse T2-weighted image represented histologically confirmed cellular periosteal reaction that could not be appreciated on radiographs or CT examination. Feathery increased signal intensity edema can be appreciated in the subcutaneous fat and muscle on the transverse T2-weighted image.

MR is likely to play an increasingly important role in the evaluation of osteomyelitis in children. In this case, MR was used to diagnose the osteomyelitis (radiographic findings were subtle and bone scan was not diagnostic) and to guide the orthopedic surgeon in his drainage procedure. The surgeon was able to make a small anterior incision in the calf and drain the largest pockets of pus. The cortical breakthrough seen on the coronal image was confirmed at surgery.

In chronic osteomyelitis, bony sclerosis is a more common finding. Sinus tracks can be identified (3), and sequestra may be seen as focal areas of low signal intensity. Prospective studies comparing MR and scintigraphic studies, particularly MDP bone scan, have not yet been done.

References

1. Modic MT, Pflanze W, Feiglin DHI, Belhobek G. Magnetic resonance imaging of musculoskeletal infections. *Radiol Clin North Am* 1986;24:247–258.
2. Beltran J, Noto AM, McGhee RB, et al. Infections of the musculoskeletal system: high-field strength MR imaging. *Radiology* 1987;164:449–454.
3. Quinn SF, Murray W, Clark RA, Cochran C. MR imaging of chronic osteomyelitis. *J Comput Assist Tomogr* 1988;12:113–117.

Submitted by: Sheila G. Moore, M.D., Stanford University, Stanford, California; Rosalind B. Dietrich, M.B., Ch.B., Senior Editor.

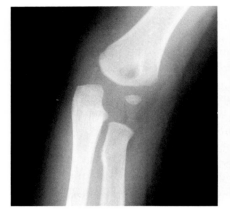

FIG. 76A.

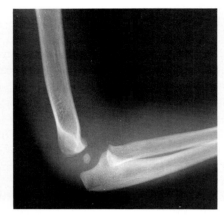

FIG. 76B.

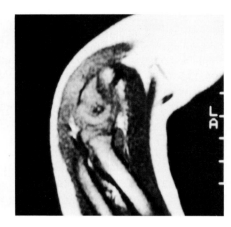

FIG. 76C. SE 300/25.

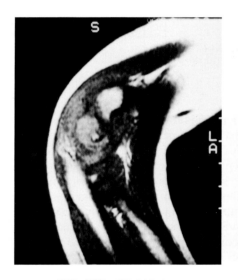

FIG. 76D. SE 300/25.

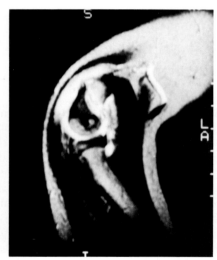

FIG. 76E. SE 2,500/70.

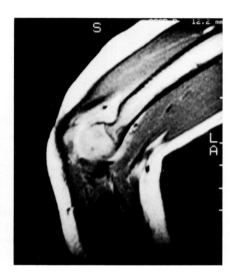

FIG. 76F. SE 2,500/20.

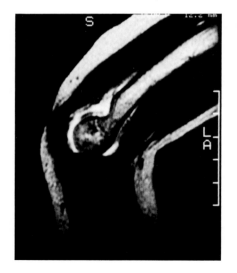

FIG. 76G. SE 2,500/70.

Clinical History

A 2-year-old boy status post-fall from tricycle, with pain and decreased motion in the right elbow.

Findings

Anteroposterior and lateral radiograph of the right elbow shows displacement of the ossified capitellum (Figs. 76A and B). No definite metaphyseal abnormality identified. No definite posterior fat pad sign is seen. Although this was likely to represent a fracture, it was uncertain whether this represented a partial fracture through the physis or a fracture involving both the metaphysis and physis (Salter II fracture). The status of the cartilaginous epiphyseal ossification centers cannot be determined on the radiograph.

Sagittal T1-W image (SE 300/25) through the elbow reveals a fracture through the physis and cartilaginous metaphysis in the distal humerus, making this a Salter II fracture of the cartilaginous distal humerus (Fig. 76C). The ossified capitellum can be appreciated as a small increased signal intensity focus with a low signal intensity rim within the cartilaginous humeral epiphysis.

The adjacent sagittal T1-W image (SE 300/25) shows the ossified capitellum to better advantage within the cartilaginous fracture fragment (Fig. 76D). The increased signal intensity fatty marrow of the distal humeral metaphysis can be appreciated just superior to the cartilaginous epiphysis. The separation of the metaphyseal fragment and capitellar epiphysis from the humeral shaft can be appreciated.

T2-W image (SE 2,500/70) through the same level as Fig. 76C. The cartilaginous metaphyseal fragment, cartilaginous epiphysis, and ossified capitellum can be appreciated as displaced from the bony humerus. Increased signal intensity blood and fluid within the joint capsule can be appreciated.

Sagittal intermediate-weighted (SE 2,500/20) and T2-W images (SE 2,500/70) through the lateral trochlear cartilaginous epiphysis (Figs. 76F and G) reveal an intact trochlear cartilaginous epiphysis, with no evidence of fracture extending through the trochlear portion of the humeral epiphysis. The low signal intensity physis can be appreciated on both images and is seen to be intact. Blood and fluid are again appreciated in the joint capsule. Because there is no ossified trochlear component to the trochlear epiphysis at this age, this information could not be obtained from the plain film.

Diagnosis

Salter II fracture of the medial (capitellar) aspect of the distal humerus epiphysis. The humeral shaft can be appreciated as intact.

Discussion

It is likely that MR will be increasingly used in the evaluation of pediatric elbow injuries. The ability to recognize cartilaginous structures on MR as well as the availability of direct coronal, axial, and sagittal images make MR theoretically superior to all other imaging modalities. MR can be used to identify fractures through cartilaginous structures that would otherwise be missed on plain film radiography; in this case recognition of the metaphyseal component of the fracture made this a Salter II and not a Salter I fracture. Perhaps most important for the surgeon, the absence of injury to cartilaginous structures such as the trochlear, medial, and lateral epiphysis obviated the need for exploration of the joint during surgery and allowed a more focused surgical correction with improved cosmetic effect.

Reference

1. Berger P. Trauma and mechanical disorders. In: Cohen MD, Edwards MK, eds. *Magnetic Resonance Imaging in Children.* Philadelphia: B. C. Decker, 1990, pp. 926–944.

Submitted by: Sheila G. Moore, M.D., Stanford University, Stanford, California; Rosalind B. Dietrich, M.B., Ch.B., Senior Editor.

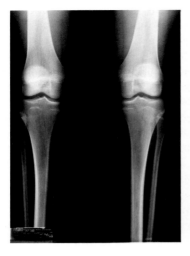

FIG. 77A.

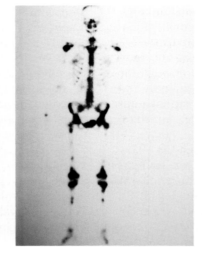

FIG. 77B.

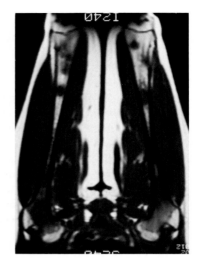

FIG. 77C. SE 300/15.

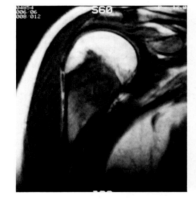

FIG. 77D. SE 300/20.

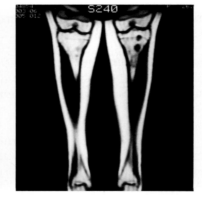

FIG. 77E. SE 300/15.

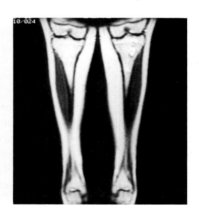

FIG. 77F. SE 2,500/80.

Clinical History

An 11-year-old girl with a 6-month history of bilateral leg pain.

Findings

Radiograph of the knees reveals no definite abnormality (Fig. 77A). Anterior technetium 99m bone scan shows multiple skeletal lesions (Fig. 77B).

Coronal T1-W image (SE 300/15) through the femurs reveals multiple low signal intensity medullary lesions (Fig. 77C). Lesions are well defined and seen throughout the metaphyseal and diaphyseal marrow. On T2-weighted images, these low signal intensity lesions were increased in signal intensity.

Coronal T1-W image (SE 300/20) through the proximal right humerus in the same patient (Fig. 77D). A low signal intensity lesion can be appreciated in the proximal metaphysis, abutting the epiphysis and extending into the fatty epiphyseal marrow.

Coronal T1-W (SE 300/15) and T2-W (SE 2,500/80) images through the tibias show multiple well-defined focal low signal intensity lesions that increase in signal intensity on the T2-weighted image (Figs. 77E and F). There is no surrounding marrow edema.

Diagnosis

Primitive neuroectodermal tumor of bone.

Discussion

Primary neuroectodermal tumors of the peripheral skeleton are rare and histologically resemble neuroectodermal tumors of the peripheral soft tissues and Ewing's sarcoma. They belong to the group of small round cell tumors that includes rhabdomyosarcoma, lymphoma, Ewing's sarcoma, and neuroblastoma. Initially described by Askin et al. (1) as tumors of neuroectodermal origin arising from thoracopulmonary soft tissues in children and adolescents, these primary neuroectodermal tumors of bone were described and redefined by Jaffe et al. in 1984 (2). The age, male predominance, and length of time between diagnosis and death are similar to that of Ewing's sarcoma; however, metastatic disease is three times more frequent at the time of the initial presentation in neuroectodermal tumors than in Ewing's sarcoma (3).

There have been no published studies of the MR appearance of the neuroectodermal tumor of bone. My experience with the tumor indicates that they may be either homogeneous, as in this case, or slightly more heterogeneous, especially when located in the ribs. Edema has not been a significant finding on the MR examinations. In a child of this age with multiple bony lesions and a biopsy that shows small round cell tumor, primary neuroectodermal tumor should be considered high in the differential. Although neuroblastoma metastatic to bone can have this identical appearance, this child's age would almost preclude that diagnosis. There is no soft tissue mass to suggest rhabdomyosarcoma. Because multiple metastatic lesions are more common in the primary neuroectodermal tumors than in Ewing's sarcoma, primary neuroectodermal tumor should lead the differential diagnosis.

Figure 77D illustrates an important point when interpreting MR images of the marrow. The ossified epiphysis always has the MR appearance of yellow marrow, even in the youngest child. Low signal intensity within the ossified epiphysis should always be considered abnormal, and the adjacent marrow should be scrutinized for abnormality. In this case, one can appreciate breakthrough of the tumor from the metaphyseal region through the physis and into the epiphysis.

References

1. Askin FB, Rosai J, Sibley PK, et al. Malignant small cell tumor of the thoracopulmonary region in childhood: a distinctive clinicopathological entity of uncertain histogenesis. *Cancer* 1979;43:2438.
2. Jaffe R, Santamaria M, Yunis EJ, et al. The neuroectodermal tumor of bone. *Am J Surg Pathol* 1984;8:885.
3. Moore SG, Dawson KL. Tumors of the musculoskeletal system. In: Cohen MD, Edwards MK, *Magnetic Resonance Imaging of Children.* Philadelphia: B. C. Decker, 1990, pp. 825–913.

Submitted by: Sheila G. Moore, M.D., Stanford University, Stanford, California; Rosalind B. Dietrich, M.B., Ch.B., Senior Editor.

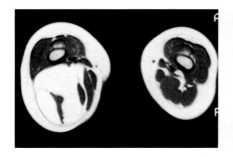

FIG. 78A. SE 800/20.

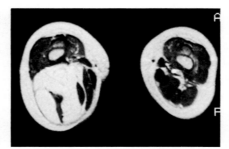

FIG. 78B. SE 2,000/80.

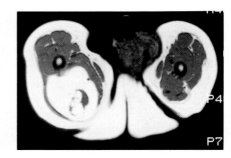

FIG. 78C. SE 800/20.

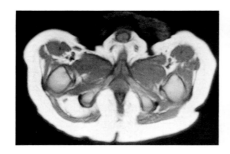

FIG. 78D. SE 800/20.

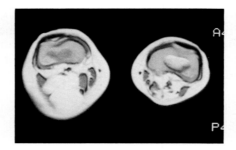

FIG. 78E. SE 2,000/20.

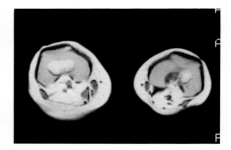

FIG. 78F. SE 2,000/20.

Clinical History

A 10-month-old boy with a right thigh mass.

Findings

Axial T1-W (SE 800/20) (Fig. 78A) and T2-W (SE 2,000/80) (Fig. 78B) images through the mid-thigh show an increased signal intensity mass intercalating around and between the muscles of the posterior thigh. The signal intensity of the mass decreases on the T2-weighted image and mirrors that of subcutaneous fat and therefore represents a fatty tumor. On the T1-weighted image, it is unclear whether the intermediate signal intensity soft tissue within the mass represents normal muscle or abnormal soft tissue. On the T2-weighted image, however, the tissue remains of intermediate signal intensity, identical to muscle, and in fact does represent muscle that is distorted and displaced by the fatty mass. Tumor or abnormal tissue would be seen as increased signal intensity on the T2-weighted image.

Axial T1-W images (SE 800/20) (Figs. 78C and D) through the proximal thigh and pelvis reveal the proximal extent of the lesion. Again, normal muscle is distorted and displaced, and the signal intensity of the mass is identical to that of the subcutaneous tissue.

Axial intermediate-weighted image (SE 2,000/20) through the distal femoral epiphysis shows the inferior extent of the fatty tumor, identified in the politeal fossa. Notice the normal appearance of the distal femoral epiphysis in a pediatric patient. On the left side, one can identify the cartilaginous distal epiphysis surrounding the ossified distal femoral epiphysis, which is seen as an increased signal intensity focus within the cartilaginous epiphysis. The increase signal intensity of the ossified femoral epiphysis reflects the yellow marrow within the ossifying epiphysis. On the right (Fig. 78E), the low signal intensity identified within the cartilaginous femoral distal epiphysis reflects a partial volume effect of the superior aspect of the ossifying epiphysis. The appearance of the normal, cartilaginous patella, seen on the left (Fig. 78F), should be noted.

Diagnosis

Lipoma of the left thigh.

Discussion

Lipomas are benign soft tissue tumors comprised of an accumulation of typical fat cells. They tend to occur in the trunk, proximal upper extremity, and thigh. They are multiple in 5% of cases. Usually encapsulated and well defined, they can rarely present as a diffuse increase in the adipose tissue with separation of muscular bundles by thick layers and masses of hyperplastic fat, as seen in this case. They can contain numerous fibrous septa. The primary differential in the pediatric patient includes diffuse lipomatosis; however, in these cases, hyperplasia of the soft tissues and bones of the affected limb is often seen. The MR appearance of lipoma and lipomatous tumors has been reported (1–4). Typically, the lipoma will be seen as a well-defined circumscribed lesion with a signal intensity identical to that of fat. Septations within lesions can be prominent, but there is typically a lack of surrounding edema. This differs from the MR appearance of the typical liposarcoma, which will likely be seen as any soft tissue tumor, intermediate signal intensity on the T1-weighted image, and increased signal intensity on the T2-weighted image. Fatty signal intensity can be seen within liposarcomas; the amount of appreciable fatty image on the MR signal can range from no appreciable fatty signal to dominant fatty signal. However, at least some "soft tissue" component should be identified. Invasion of surrounding muscle and soft tissue planes, as well as surrounding edema, would also support the diagnosis of liposarcoma rather than lipoma.

References

1. Totty WG, Murphy WA, Lee JKT. Soft-tissue tumors: MR imaging. *Radiology* 1986;160:135–141.
2. Kransdorf MJ, Jelinek JS, Moser RP Jr, et al. Soft-tissue masses: diagnosis using MR imaging. *AJR* 1989;153:541–547.
3. Dooms GC, Hricak H, Solitto RA, Higgins CB. Lipomatous tumors and tumors with fatty component: MR imaging potential and comparison of MR and CT results. *Radiology* 1985;157:479–483.
4. Moore SG, Dawson KL. Tumors of the musculoskeletal system. In: Cohen MD, ed. *Pediatric MRI*. Philadelphia: B. C. Decker (*In press*).

Submitted by: Sheila G. Moore, M.D., Stanford University, Stanford, California; Rosalind B. Dietrich, M.B., Ch.B., Senior Editor.

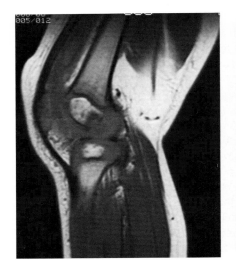

FIG. 79A. SE 800/20.

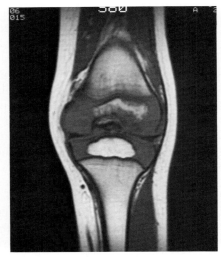

FIG. 79B. SE 800/20.

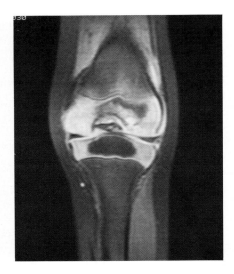

FIG. 79C. SE 2,000/20 with spectroscopic fat suppression.

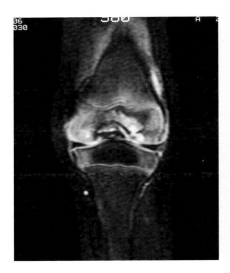

FIG. 79D. SE 2,000/80 with spectroscopic fat suppression.

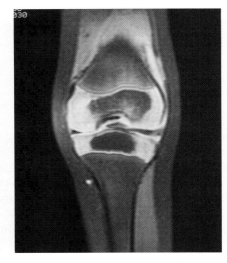

FIG. 79E. SE 2,000/20 with spectroscopic fat suppression.

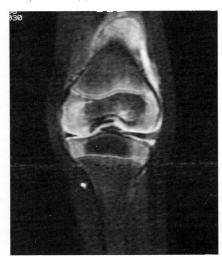

FIG. 79F. SE 2,000/80 with spectroscopic fat suppression.

Clinical History

A 2-year-old boy with a 2-week history of left knee pain and swelling.

Findings

Sagittal T1-W image (SE 800/20) through the left knee revealed a defect in the ossified distal femoral epiphysis posteriorly (Fig. 79A). Close inspection shows subtle decreased signal intensity that is lower than that of surrounding cartilaginous epiphysis. Subtle decreased signal intensity is seen in the distal femoral metaphysis, adjacent to the physis. Low signal intensity is appreciated within the suprapatella bursa, consistent with effusion.

Coronal T1-W image (SE 800/20) through the knee reveals a normal tibial shaft and normal ossified tibial epiphysis (Fig. 79B). The normal cartilaginous tibial epiphysis can be seen surrounding the ossified epiphysis. In the femur, an intermediate signal intensity defect is again seen in the posterior aspect of the ossified distal femoral epiphysis. The cartilaginous distal femoral epiphysis can be appreciated, and again subtle decreased signal intensity is seen in the distal femoral metaphysis adjacent to the physis.

Intermediate-weighted (SE 2,000/20) (Fig. 79C) and T2-W (SE 2,000/80) (Fig. 79D) fat saturation images at the same level as Fig. 79B. The suppressed yellow marrow of the tibial shaft and ossified tibial epiphysis can be appreciated. A focal, increased signal intensity lesion can be seen within the ossified femoral epiphysis (with suppressed fatty marrow signals seen surrounding the increased signal intensity lesion). The increased signal intensity lesion extends into the cartilaginous femoral epiphysis (cf. Fig. 79B). Note the increased signal intensity marrow in the distal femoral metaphysis adjacent to the physis. Cartilaginous structures are normally seen as increased signal intensity, as illustrated in the tibial epiphysis. Increased signal intensity fluid is appreciated lateral and anterior to the femoral metaphysis.

Diagnosis

Acute staphylococcal osteomyelitis of the left distal femoral epiphysis, cartilaginous and ossified portions.

Discussion

Early diagnosis of osteomyelitis is essential in preventing the complications of delayed or inadequate treatment. Risk factors include systemic disease, immunosuppression, and traumatic injury.

Although osteomyelitis in children is typically described as a metaphyseal lesion, we are seeing increasing numbers of patients with biopsy-proven epiphyseal osteomyelitis identified on MR images. This includes osteomyelitis in both the ossified and cartilaginous epiphysis. On MR images, acute osteomyelitis is usually seen as decreased signal intensity on T1-weighted images and normal or increased signal intensity on T2-weighted images (1,2). Surrounding soft tissue edema and inflammation are a common component. If the infection is in the joint, complex joint effusion is usually seen.

This case demonstrates the usefulness of T2-weighted fat saturation images (3). Fat signal suppression is achieved by a frequency-selective 90-degree pulse at the frequency of the lipid methylene proton signal just prior to the 90-degree pulse of the spin-echo sequence. This results in the lipid methylene protons being tipped by approximately 180 degrees, whereas the water protons are tipped 90 degrees by the first pulse of the spin-echo sequence (3). Lipid signal is therefore suppressed, resulting in an enhanced T2-weighted image. The advantage of this imaging sequence when compared to other techniques such as short TI inversion recovery imaging is that more slices can be obtained with either the same or a decreased acquisition time.

References

1. Modic MT, Pflanze W, Feiglin DHI, Belhobek G. Magnetic resonance imaging of musculoskeletal infections. *Radiol Clin North Am* 1986;24:247–258.
2. Beltran J, Noto AM, McGhee RB, et al. Infections of the musculoskeletal system: high-field strength MR imaging. *Radiology* 1987;164:449–454.
3. Block RE, Parekh BC. Enhanced proton magnetic resonance imaging of experimental mammary tumors. *Magn Reson Med* 1988;6:116–118.

Submitted by: Sheila G. Moore, M.D., Stanford University, Stanford, California; Rosalind B. Dietrich, M.B., Ch.B., Senior Editor.

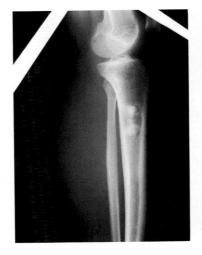

FIG. 80A.

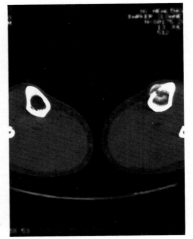

FIG. 80B. CT.

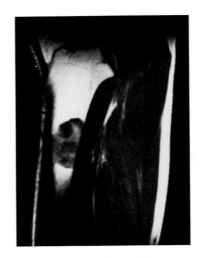

FIG. 80C. SE 800/20.

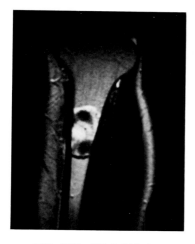

FIG. 80D. SE 2,000/80.

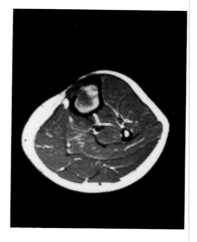

FIG. 80E. SE 900/20.

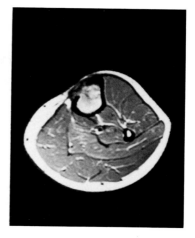

FIG. 80F. SE 2,000/20.

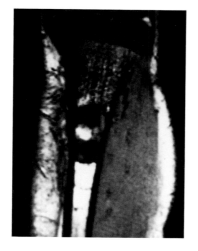

FIG. 80G. GRE 60/40/30°.

Clinical History

A 25-year-old male with a 6-month history of left tibial pain.

Findings

Lateral radiograph of the left tibia shows a complex lesion in the proximal tibial metaphysis with both a lytic and blastic component (Fig. 80A).

Axial CT scan through the tibias reveals a lytic and blastic medullary lesion in the proximal tibial metaphysis (Fig. 80B). Cortical breakthrough of the anteromedial surface of the tibia is noted, with blastic bone present in the surrounding soft tissues.

Sagittal T1-W image (SE 800/20) through the left tibia shows a well-defined, heterogeneous signal intensity lesion in the tibial metaphysis (Fig. 80C).

Coronal T2-W image (SE 2,000/80) through the tibia again shows the heterogeneous increased signal intensity lesion within the tibial marrow (Fig. 80D). Note the foci of low signal intensity. This corresponds to blastic bone and is a hallmark of blastic osteogenic sarcoma.

T1-W (SE 900/20) (Fig. 80E) and intermediate-weighted (SE 2,000/20) (Fig. 80F) axial images through the lesion. Breakthrough of the tumor through the cortical bone can be appreciated on both images. The inter-mediate signal intensity tumor appreciated on the T1-weighted image is seen as increased signal intensity on the T2-weighted image.

Coronal gradient recalled echo image (GRE 60/40, 30 degrees) through the tibia (Fig. 80G) at a level similar to that of Fig. 80D. The inferior margin of the lesion is well defined and easily appreciated when compared to the increased signal intensity fatty marrow in the diaphysis. However, the superior margin of the lesion is less well defined on this image. This is due to the magnetic susceptibility effect of trabecular bone on surrounding marrow signal intensity in the metaphysis and epiphysis. Compared to Fig. 80D, regions seen as low signal intensity blastic bone on the T2-weighted image are also seen as low signal intensity blastic bone on the GRE image. The central region of the tumor seen as increased signal intensity on the T2-weighted image is also seen as increased signal intensity on the gradient echo image. This indicates lack of trabecular bone and corresponds to a lytic lesion.

Diagnosis

Osteogenic sarcoma.

Discussion

Osteogenic sarcoma is the most common primary bone tumor in children. It arises primarily from undifferentiated connective tissue of bone that forms neoplastic osteoid in osseous tissue (1). It is a disease of older children and young adults. Eighty-six percent of lesions are seen in the long bones, with a majority of these located around the knee joint. The gross histologic appearance, and to some degree the MR appearance, of the tumor will depend on the predominant type of tumor tissue present. Osteosarcomas are classified as osteoblastic, chondroblastic, fibroblastic, or telangiectatic. On radiographs, the tumors are usually either sclerotic or lytic in type, although many tumors will have a component of both sclerosis and lysis. The degree of sclerosis or blastic bone seen on plain film reflects the amounts of osteoid, tumor bone, and reactive bone within the lesion. In general, this new bone or reactive bone formation will be seen as low signal intensity on both T1- and T2-weighted MR images. The more cellular portions of the tumors will be seen as intermediate signal intensity on T1-weighted images and increased signal intensity on T2-weighted images. Therefore, a lesion that is seen in a child or young adult, around the knee joint, that consists of signal intensities suggesting both cellular and blastic bone components is likely to represent an osteogenic sar-coma. Other tumors can cause reactive bone formation, and, as always, the radiograph must be compared to the MR examination to assist in distinguishing osteogenic sarcoma from other bone lesions.

MRI following plain radiograph is considered by many to be the imaging method of choice in the diagnosis, staging, and follow-up of osteogenic sarcoma. In addition to identification of the medullary extent of the tumor, MRI is useful to evaluate for cortical involvement, cortical breakthrough (as seen in this case), and surrounding soft tissue involvement.

GRE imaging is currently being used more frequently in clinical imaging of the musculoskeletal system. It is therefore important that one understands the marrow contrast seen on GRE imaging. The marrow signal seen on GRE imaging reflects primarily the amount of trabecular bone present within that particular marrow space (2). Magnetic susceptibility effects in the marrow caused by the presence of trabecular bone within the marrow cause a decrement of signal intensity on GRE images that reflects the amount of trabecular bone present. Therefore, those regions of bone with a large amount of trabecular bone (epiphysis, patella) show a loss of signal intensity when compared to those regions of marrow with little or no trabecular bone (diaphysis) (Fig. 80G).

Thus, as in this case, fatty marrow within the tibial epiphysis is seen as low signal intensity, or black, whereas fatty marrow within the diaphysis is seen as bright signal intensity (the expected signal intensity on a spin-echo image). The blastic bone within the tumor enhances this susceptibility effect and is seen as black on the GRE image. The lytic region of the tumor is seen as bright signal intensity, since the magnetic susceptibility effect caused by trabecular bone is absent.

References

1. Moore SG, Dawson KL. Tumors of the musculoskeletal system. In: Cohen MD, Edwards MK, ed. *Magnetic Resonance Imaging of Children.* Philadelphia: B. C. Decker, 1990, pp. 825–913.
2. Sebag GH, Moore SG. Effect of trabecular bone on the appearance of marrow in gradient echo imaging of the appendicular skeleton. *Radiology (in press).*

Submitted by: Sheila G. Moore, M.D., Stanford University, Stanford, California; Rosalind B. Dietrich, M.B., Ch.B., Senior Editor.

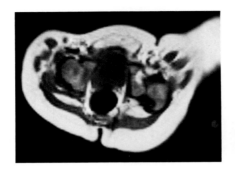

FIG. 81A. SE 1,000/40.

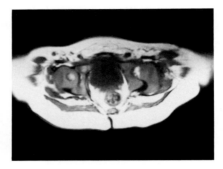

FIG. 81B. SE 600/20. 4 months after 81A with patient in spice cast.

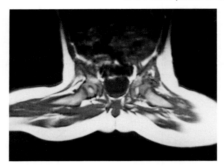

FIG. 81C. SE 600/20. 4 months after 81A with patient in spice cast.

Clinical History

A 9-month-old boy with suspected congenital dislocation of the hip (CDH).

Findings

Axial T1-W image (SE 1,000/40) through the acetabulae shows the cartilaginous femoral head on the right well seated within the right acetabulum (Fig. 81A). On the left, the acetabulum is well formed, but the cartilaginous femoral head is posteriorly displaced with respect to the acetabulum. Increased signal intensity fatty pulvinar is present within the acetabulum.

Axial T1-W image (SE 600/20) of the acetabulae 4 months after the patient was placed in a spica cast (Fig. 81B). The examination is performed with the spica cast on the patient. The right femoral head is well seated within the normal acetabulum, and the increased signal intensity ossified femoral epiphysis is seen centrally within the cartilaginous femoral epiphysis. On the left, the acetabulum can be identified, but the femoral head does not appear to be well seated within the acetabulum. Increased signal intensity fatty pulvinar can be seen interposed between the acetabulum and the cartilaginous head. There is no identifiable ossified femoral epiphysis.

Coronal T1-W image (SE 600/20) taken with the patient in the spica cast shows the normal relationship of the right femoral head to the right acetabulum (Fig. 81C). On the left, however, superior and lateral subluxation of the cartilaginous femoral head in relationship to the acetabulum can be appreciated.

Diagnosis

Superoposterior congenital dislocation of left hip and persistent subluxation of the left femoral head despite closed reduction and spica cast treatment.

Discussion

Although dynamic ultrasonography is likely to play an increasingly important role in the initial evaluation of the neonate or infant with suspected CDH, MR will likely play an increasingly important role in the evaluation of the older child with CDH or the child requiring prolonged treatment for CDH. The advantages of dynamic ultrasonography in the evaluation of CDH include widespread availability, lack of ionizing radiation, and relatively low cost. The disadvantages include operator dependence, the potential lack of acceptance on the part of referring physicians and orthopedic surgeons, and the inability to easily image the patient once he or she has been placed in a spica cast. Although MR can be costly, it is possible that a screening examination consisting of T1-weighted axial and coronal images may become a cost-effective modality in evaluating the complicated or long-term patient with CDH. Certainly, the use of ultrasonography and MR is preferable to the use of radiographs and CT, in which ionizing radiation directed at the evaluation of the hips results in gonadal irradiation.

Because MR images readily reflect cartilaginous structures, MR evaluation accurately and reliably allows visualization of the cartilaginous structures of the hip, so that exact anatomic relationships can be determined. MR has a potential role in the identification and evaluation of inverted limbus and hourglass capsule, which may in the future obviate the need for hip arthrography in the older or complicated patient with CDH.

Reference

1. Johnson ND, Wood BP, Jackman KV. Complex infantile and congenital hip dislocation: assessment with MR imaging. *Radiology* 1988;168:151.

Submitted by: Sheila G. Moore, M.D., Stanford University, Stanford, California; Rosalind B. Dietrich, M.B., Ch.B., Senior Editor.

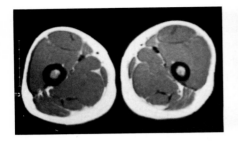 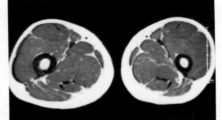 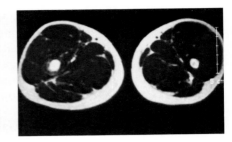

FIG. 82A. SE 600/15.   FIG. 82B. SE 2,000/30.   FIG. 82C. SE 2,000/75.

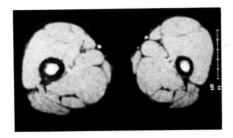 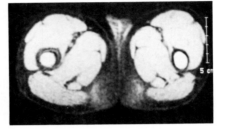

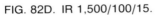

FIG. 82D. IR 1,500/100/15.   FIG. 82E. IR 1,500/100/15.

Clinical History

A 5-year-old boy with treated neuroblastoma presenting with new onset right hip and femur pain.

Findings

Axial T1-W image (SE 600/15) through the proximal femurs reveals intermediate signal intensity within expanded cortical bone in the right femoral shaft (Fig. 82A). The signal intensity of the marrow is intermediate bilaterally.

Axial intermediate-weighted (SE 2,000/30) and T2-W (SE 2,000/75) images through the same level show a persistence of intermediate (Fig. 82B) and increased (Fig. 82C) signal intensity within the expanded cortical bone on the right. The signal intensity of the marrow bilaterally is bright on both the intermediate and T2-weighted images and can be appreciated as brighter than the subcutaneous fat on the T2-weighted image.

Transverse short TI inversion recovery (STIR) image (IR 1,500/100/15) at the same level as the spin-echo images (Fig. 82D). The increased signal intensity within the right cortical bone can be appreciated, as can the increased signal intensity in the marrow in the femoral shafts bilaterally.

Diagnosis

Diffuse metastatic neuroblastoma to the femurs.

Discussion

Femoral biopsy confirmed the presence of metastatic neuroblastoma in the femurs. Intermediate signal intensity within cortical bone is not normal and should be recognized. This finding is illustrated in the right femur. When seen, it may correspond to periosteal reaction on plain film, and in this case lamellated periosteal reaction was identified. Periosteal reaction can be identified on MR images (1) and should be assessed. When cortical abnormality is seen, close inspection of the adjacent bone marrow is warranted.

In general, the signal intensity of the marrow of the femoral diaphysis on spin-echo images will be that of fatty marrow in children over the age of 5 years (2). In fact, on coronal images, the femoral diaphyseal shaft will usually appear as increased signal intensity on T1-weighted images in children over the age of 1 or 2 years. The presence of intermediate signal intensity marrow in the femoral diaphysis on T1-weighted images should prompt close inspection of the signal intensity of the marrow on T2-weighted and fat suppression or STIR images. If the marrow signal intensity is intermediate on T1-weighted images and appears brighter than that of subcutaneous fat on the T2-weighted image, infiltration of the marrow by abnormal cells is likely. The other possibility to be considered in these instances is reconversion of the normal fatty marrow to hematopoietic marrow under conditions of marrow stress. This can be seen in children with chronic anemias, i.e., thalassemia or sickle cell anemia, and can also be seen in response to chemotherapy. The extent of abnormality and the patient's history and clinical status can aid in determining the etiology of the marrow abnormality.

Both STIR and T2 fat suppression images are useful in the evaluation of pediatric marrow. However, caution must be used when interpreting these images, because normal hematopoietic marrow can be seen as increased signal intensity in both of these imaging sequences. In general, hematopoietic marrow will be seen as intermediate to slightly increased signal intensity on STIR and T2 fat suppression images, whereas abnormal cells have very bright signal intensity.

References

1. Moore SG, Sebag GH, Dawson KL. MR evaluation of cortical bone and periosteal reaction in bone lesions: pathologic and radiographic correlation. Book of Abstracts, Society of Magnetic Resonance in Medicine 1989;1:19.
2. Moore SG, Dawson KL. Red and yellow marrow in the femur: age related changes in appearance at MR imaging. *Radiology* (in press).

Submitted by: Sheila G. Moore, M.D., Stanford University, Stanford, California; Rosalind B. Dietrich, M.B., Ch.B., Senior Editor.

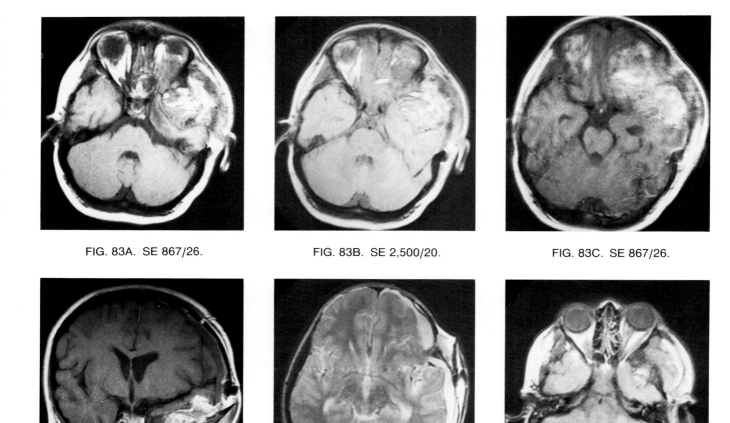

FIG. 83A. SE 867/26.

FIG. 83B. SE 2,500/20.

FIG. 83C. SE 867/26.

FIG. 83D. SE 867/26.

FIG. 83E. SE 2,500/80.

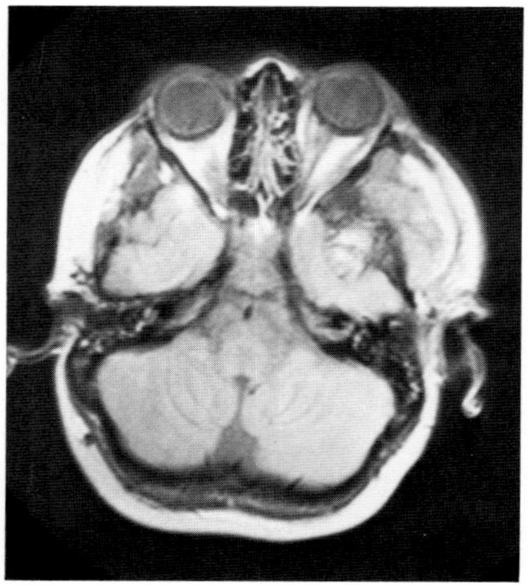

FIG. 83F. SE 2,500/20.

Clinical History

A 7-year-old boy with a history of headaches.

Findings

There is a very large mass lesion on the left side of the skull. It involves the lateral wall and roof of the left orbit, the greater wing of the left sphenoid bone, and the left parietal and temporal bones. The intracranial soft tissue component is causing elevation and displacement of the left frontal and temporal lobes (Figs. 83A–D). There is extension medially over the roof of the orbit close to the cribriform plate. There is invasion of the orbit; the extraconal mass causes medial displacement of the lateral rectus muscle and mild proptosis (Fig. 83F). The mild elevation of the parietal bone and the adjacent subdural and subgaleal fluid collections (Fig. 83E) are the result of a small biopsy performed 6 days previously.

Diagnosis

Ewing's sarcoma of the skull.

Discussion

Ewing's sarcoma is a small, round cell tumor with peak incidence at approximately 8–15 years of age. It usually occurs in the peripheral skeleton but can occasionally arise in the skull. The MR images show a large mass lesion with bone involvement but without clear invasion of brain. The lesion shows increase in signal intensity with T2 weighting and enhancement following gadolinium administration. The appearance of the lesion is very nonhomogeneous, and this, together with some high signal intensity seen on the T1-weighted image (Fig. 83A), may be due to hemorrhage within the tumor.

The differential diagnosis would include osteomyelitis with adjacent abscess and histiocytosis. Primary bone lymphoma is another consideration, although the large soft tissue component would be unusual for lymphoma. Metastasis from neuroblastoma might look like this lesion; however, the patient is slightly older than the peak incidence for neuroblastoma (but still within the accepted age range).

References

1. Boyko OB, et al. MR imaging of osteogenic and Ewing sarcoma. *AJR* 1987;148:317–322.
2. Bloem JL, et al. Radiologic staging of primary bone sarcoma: MR imaging, scintigraphy, angiography and CT correlated with pathologic examination. *Radiology* 1988;169:805–810.
3. Bloem JL, et al. Magnetic resonance imaging of primary malignant bone tumors. *RadioGraphics* 1987;7:425–445.

Submitted by: Mervyn D. Cohen, M.B., Ch.B., Riley Hospital for Children, Indiana University Medical Center, Indianapolis, Indiana; Rosalind B. Dietrich, M.B., Ch.B., Senior Editor.

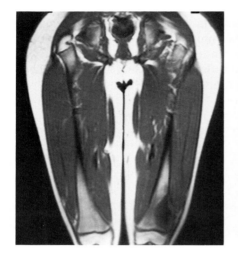

FIG. 84A. SE 667/20.

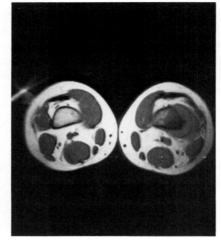

FIG. 84B. SE 800/20.

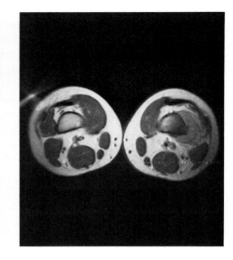

FIG. 84C. SE 800/20.

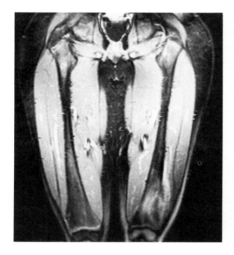

FIG. 84D. IR 2,000/150/30.

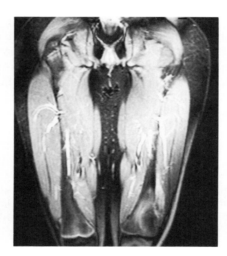

FIG. 84E. IR 2,000/150/30.

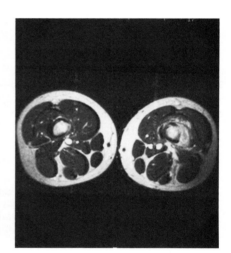

FIG. 84F. SE 2,000/80.

Clinical History

A 12-year-old white male with a 1-month history of pain in the distal thigh with increasing discomfort on walking.

Findings

Figures 84A and B are coronal and axial T1-weighted images. There is a well-defined abnormality involving the distal left femoral metaphysis with extension into the soft tissue. There is a fairly well-defined interface between normal and abnormal bone marrow. The lesion appears to penetrate the lateral cortex with a small adjacent soft tissue mass. A few very low intensity spots seen in the soft tissue mass on the axial image represent calcium. The lesion extends up to but does not appear to cross the growth plate. The knee joint appears normal. Following gadolinium administration (Fig. 84C), there is minimal increase in signal intensity in the soft tissue component of the tumor with little, if any, change in the appearance of the diseased bone marrow. Short TI inversion recovery (STIR) pulse sequences (Figs. 84D and E) show an area of abnormality similar to that seen on the coronal T1-weighted image. The low signal intensity represents calcification and new bone formation. The extent of the lesion in the soft tissue and bone marrow corresponds fairly well to the overall extent seen on the plain film radiograph. Of interest is the abnormal high signal intensity in both the distal femoral and proximal tibial epiphyses on the left. T2-weighted image (Fig. 84F) shows increase in signal intensity of both the soft tissue and bone marrow components of the lesion. At other levels, many areas of the lesion do not increase in signal intensity due to calcification and new bone formation.

Diagnosis

Osteogenic sarcoma, blastic type. The abnormal signal in the distal femoral and proximal tibial epiphysis on the STIR pulse sequence is believed to be due to reactive traumatic edema and not to tumor invasion.

Discussion

Osteogenic sarcomas are the most common primary bone tumors in children, occurring most commonly in patients between the ages of 10 and 25 years. More than 80% of lesions occur in the long bones, and the most common location is around the knee joint. They most commonly arise in the metaphysis and may spread into the diaphysis or across the growth plate into the epiphysis and even into the adjacent joint. With most osteogenic sarcomas MR demonstrates much more extensive bone marrow spread than would be anticipated from the plain film radiograph. With the less common blastic type of osteogenic sarcoma, the overall extent of abnormality in the marrow, demonstrated on MR, usually corresponds closely to the extent of abnormality seen on plain film. MR can demonstrate penetration of cortex, seen as increase in the normal very low intensity signal from the cortex. Periosteal reaction can be appreciated but not as easily as on the plain film radiograph.

The MR findings of osteogenic sarcoma are somewhat nonspecific. MR always demonstrates involvement of the bone marrow, cortex, and adjacent soft tissue. The bone marrow shows decreased signal intensity on T1-weighted images. The soft tissue lesion is always bright on T2 sequences. It is usually well defined and may be quite large. Optimal therapy involves resection of the tumor mass either at presentation or following a trial course of chemotherapy. MR is extremely sensitive in demonstrating the total spread of tumor within the bone marrow, and this is helpful in determining the level of surgical resection.

References

1. Cohen MD, et al. Magnetic resonance imaging of bone marrow disease in children. *Radiology* 1984;151:715–718.
2. Boyko OB, et al. Magnetic resonance imaging of osteogenic sarcoma and Ewing's sarcoma. *AJR* 1987;148:317–322.
3. Gillespy T, et al. Staging of intraosseous extent of osteosarcoma: correlation of preoperative CT and MR imaging with pathologic macroslides. *Radiology* 1988;167:765–767.
4. Jones BE, et al. MR appearances of childhood bone tumors. *AJR* 1989;153:202–203.

Submitted by: Mervyn D. Cohen, M.B., Ch.B., Riley Hospital for Children, Indiana University Medical Center, Indianapolis, Indiana; Rosalind B. Dietrich, M.B., Ch.B., Senior Editor.

CASE 85

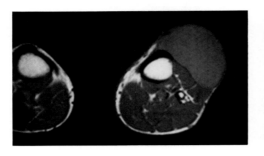 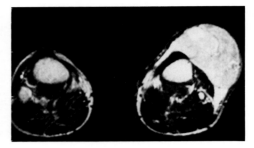

FIG. 85A. SE 800/20.   FIG. 85B. SE 2,050/90.

Clinical History

A 14-year-old black male with a history of painless swelling just below the left knee.

Findings

T1- (Fig. 85A) and T2-W (Fig. 85B) images show an extremely well-defined soft tissue mass in the anterolateral aspect of the left leg, just below the knee joint. The mass is homogeneous on the T1-weighted image with moderately uniform high signal intensity on T2-weighted images. There is very little residual overlying subcutaneous fat. There is no edema in the adjacent muscle. The adjacent cortex of the tibia is normal, and the bone marrow of both tibia and fibula appears normal.

Diagnosis

Undifferentiated soft tissue sarcoma.

Discussion

The MR appearance of many soft tissue mass lesions is nonspecific, and the final diagnosis is often not made until biopsy. MR is excellent at accurately defining the anatomic location and extent of the lesion. This may help with differential diagnosis and is extremely helpful in planning surgical resection. Most mass lesions are of intensity similar to normal muscle on T1-weighted images with increase in signal intensity on T2-weighted images. A strong signal intensity on T1-weighted image would favor the diagnosis of lipoma, hemorrhagic cyst, or fluid with a high protein content. Hemorrhage into a soft tissue lesion will cause patchy increase in signal intensity on T1-weighted images, depending on its age. A very bright signal intensity on T2-weighted image would favor the diagnosis of a fluid-filled cystic lesion. Absence of any bone involvement, as in this patient, obviously excludes bone tumor or osteomyelitis from the differential diagnosis.

References

1. Cohen MD, et al. Magnetic resonance evaluation of disease of the soft tissues in children. *Pediatrics* 1987;79:696–701.
2. Kransdorf MJ, et al. Soft tissue masses: diagnosis using MR imaging. *AJR* 1989;153:541–547.
3. Sundaram M, et al. Soft tissue masses: histologic basis for decreased signal (short T2) on T2 weighted MR images. *AJR* 1987;148:1247–1250.

Submitted by: Mervyn D. Cohen, M.B., Ch.B., Riley Hospital for Children, Indiana University Medical Center, Indianapolis, Indiana; Rosalind B. Dietrich, M.B., Ch.B., Senior Editor.

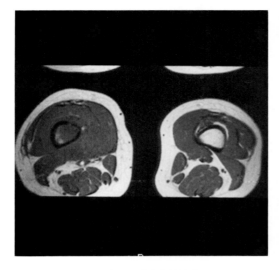

FIG. 86A. SE 717/20.

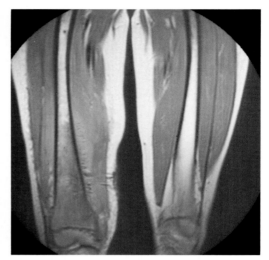

FIG. 86B. SE 2,000/20.

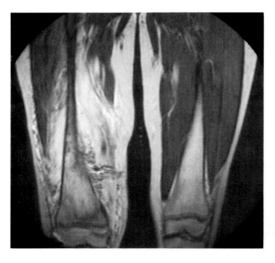

FIG. 86C. SE 2,000/80.

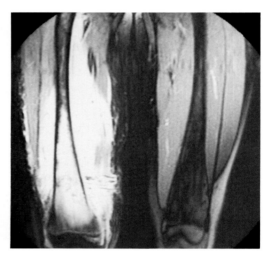

FIG. 86D. IR 2,000/150/30.

Clinical History

A 9-year-old boy with a history of poor health and intermittent pain in the right leg for several months.

Findings

Axial T1-weighted image (Fig. 86A) shows marked asymmetry of the soft tissues of the two sides. There is swelling of the muscles on the right side, with signal intensity similar to normal muscle. There is marked loss of signal intensity from the bone marrow of the right side, with some increase in signal intensity in the cortex of the right distal femur, particularly anteriorly. Coronal spin density image (Fig. 86B) shows a moderately well-defined demarcation between low intensity distal abnormal marrow and proximal normal marrow. The soft tissue swelling is again identified with minimal increase in signal intensity compared to normal muscle. T2-weighted image (Fig. 86C) and STIR pulse sequence (Fig. 86D) show a large, well-defined, soft tissue component to the lesion with very bright signal intensity. There is increase in signal intensity in the distal femur on both of these pulse sequences, more marked on the STIR sequence.

Diagnosis

Subacute osteomyelitis.

Discussion

The MR findings of osteomyelitis include abnormality affecting the bone marrow, bone cortex, and adjacent soft tissue. The soft tissues are invariably affected, and a diagnosis of osteomyelitis should seriously be doubted if the soft tissues are completely normal. The affected bone marrow and soft tissues have nonspecific signal intensities consistent with prolongation of T1 and T2 relaxation times. Cortical involvement is subtle but can usually be identified, as it was with this patient. The differentiation of acute from subacute osteomyelitis may be difficult. Features that would favor a chronic infection would be a sharp interface between normal and abnormal bone marrow, and a relatively small but well-defined soft tissue abnormality. There is, however, overlap between the different categories of osteomyelitis.

The differential diagnosis is somewhat large, and if a plain film radiograph is not obtained it may be difficult. MR and plain film findings together should allow the correct diagnosis to be made in most patients. On MR osteogenic sarcoma may appear very similar to osteomyelitis, particularly to subacute or chronic osteomyelitis, as with this patient. The margins of the soft tissue involvement in osteogenic sarcoma are usually, however, slightly better defined than with this patient. Trauma with soft tissue contusion may also appear similar. The fracture should, however, be easily diagnosed on the plain film radiograph, and the history should make the diagnosis easy.

References

1. Beltran J, et al. Infections of the musculoskeletal system: high field strength MR imaging. *Radiology* 1987;164:449–454.
2. Unger E, et al. Diagnosis of osteomyelitis by MR imaging. *AJR* 1988;150:605–610.
3. Tang JSH, et al. Musculoskeletal infection of the extremities: evaluation with MR imaging. *Radiology* 1988;166:205–209.
4. Cohen MD, et al. Magnetic resonance differentiation of acute and chronic osteomyelitis in children. *Clin Radiol* 1990;41:53–56.

Submitted by: Mervyn D. Cohen, M.B., Ch.B., Riley Hospital for Children, Indiana University Medical Center, Indianapolis, Indiana; Rosalind B. Dietrich, M.B., Ch.B., Senior Editor.

CASE 87

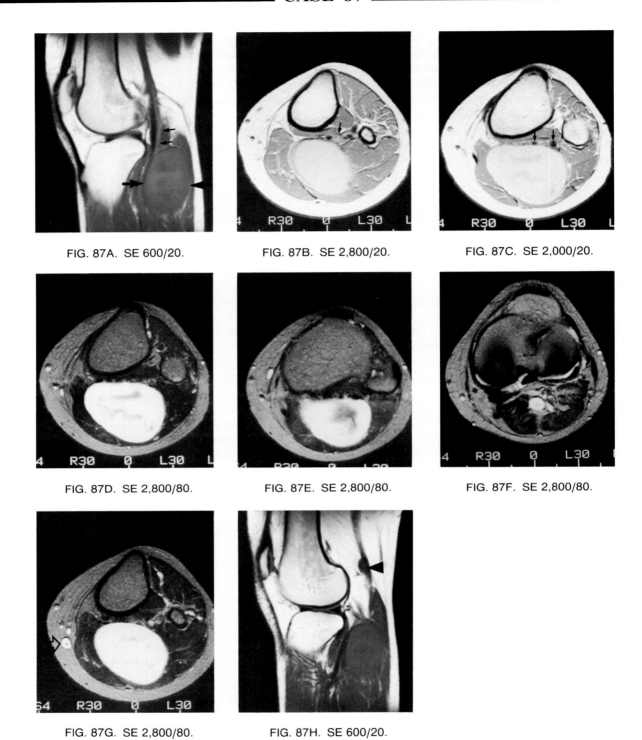

FIG. 87A. SE 600/20.

FIG. 87B. SE 2,800/20.

FIG. 87C. SE 2,000/20.

FIG. 87D. SE 2,800/80.

FIG. 87E. SE 2,800/80.

FIG. 87F. SE 2,800/80.

FIG. 87G. SE 2,800/80.

FIG. 87H. SE 600/20.

Clinical History

An 18-year-old female presented with discomfort and swelling in the left calf. She had a previous history of resection of a mass from the cervical region in early childhood. On physical examination, swelling of the left calf was noted and cutaneous abnormalities were also seen.

Findings

An MR scan of the lower limb was obtained with T1-weighted sagittal and coronal images and axial double echo images.

There is a well-defined mass, 6 × 4.5 cm (Fig. 87A, *short black arrows*) arising from the tibial nerve (Fig. 87A, *small black arrows;* Fig. 87F, *black arrow*) and extending distally within the muscles of the calf. The mass is posterior to the posterior tibial vessels (Fig. 87C, *small black arrows*). The neurovascular bundle, including the tibial nerve, is again identified distally on axial scans (Fig. 87B, *small black arrow*).

Signal intensity within the mass is inhomogeneous (Figs. 87C–F). The lesion is of generally lower signal intensity than muscle on the T1-weighted images and of high signal intensity on T2 weighting, comparable to the signal from peripheral nerve.

Additional small lesions are seen, one in the subcutaneous tissues of the proximal lower leg medially (Fig. 87G, *open arrow*) and another posteriorly in the distal thigh (Fig. 87H, *black arrowhead*).

Diagnosis

Neurofibroma arising from the tibial nerve in a patient with neurofibromatosis (NF).

Discussion

NF, together with tuberous sclerosis, and Hippel-Lindau and Sturge-Weber syndromes, constitute the phakomatoses or neurocutaneous syndromes (1). They are also referred to as congenital neuroectodermal dysplasia. However, in addition to the dysplasias and/or neoplasias of organs derived from the primitive ectoderm, structures derived from embryonic mesoderm and endoderm may be affected (1).

NF is transmitted as an autosomal dominant in approximately 50% of cases. It occurs in 30–40 persons per 100,000. NF is a dysplasia in which the neural ectodermal Schwann cell is the proliferative element with a variable degree of reactive mesenchymal hyperplasia (2).

The possible manifestations of NF are very extensive, and it can involve the CNS, skin, eye, musculoskeletal system, gastrointestinal tract, genitourinary system, lungs, and endocrine glands.

NF can be divided into central (CNF) and peripheral forms. In CNF there are usually higher morbidity and mortality (1).

The peripheral form in this patient consists of numerous nerve sheath tumors and café-au-lait spots. On MR, the schwannomas are of intermediate signal intensity on short TR sequences and are hyperintense with long TR, corresponding to the appearance of neural tissue. Contiguity with the neurovascular bundle is significant as is the presence of multiple lesions. Signal intensity within the mass may be inhomogeneous, but this does not necessarily indicate malignant change (3).

References

1. Braffman BM, Bilaniuk LT, Zimmerman RA. The central nervous system manifestations of the phakomatoses on MR. *Radiol Clin North Am* 1988;26–38.
2. Naidich TP, Zimmerman RA. Common congenital malformations of the brain. In: Brant-Zawadski M, Norman D, eds. *Magnetic resonance imaging of the central nervous system.* New York: Raven Press, 1987, pp. 131–151.
3. Levine E, Huntrakoon M, Wetzel LH. Malignant nerve sheath neoplasms in neurofibromatosis: distinction from benign tumors by using imaging techniques. *AJR* 1987;149:1059–1064.

Submitted by: Patricia E. Perry, M.D., Good Samaritan Regional Medical Center and Phoenix Children's Hospital, Phoenix, Arizona; Rosalind B. Dietrich, M.B., Ch.B., Senior Editor.

CASE 88

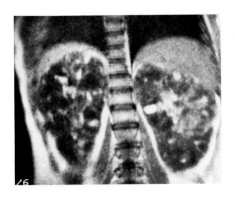

FIG. 88A. SE 1,500/56.

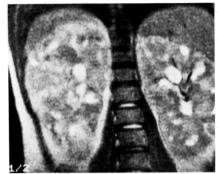

FIG. 88B. SE 1,500/56.

Clinical History

A 14-year-old girl with a history of renal failure now presents with flank pain.

Findings

MR images show massively enlarged kidneys bilaterally. There are multiple cysts present within them. Although most of the cysts have signal intensities consistent with simple cysts (low signal intensity on T1- and high signal intensity on T2-weighted images), some of the cysts demonstrate high signal intensity on both T1- and T2-weighted images.

Diagnosis

Autosomal recessive polycystic kidney disease with hemorrhage.

Discussion

Also frequently referred to as infantile polycystic disease, autosomal recessive polycystic disease is a congenital abnormality affecting both kidneys. Patients may present at varying ages and demonstrate a spectrum of pathology. Associated liver disease ranges from proliferation and dilation of the biliary radicles (biliary atresia) to severe periportal fibrosis. The severity of renal cystic disease and hepatic fibrosis varies inversely.

In infants presenting with the disease, the kidneys are greatly enlarged in size bilaterally. They contain multiple fusiform cysts, formed from dilated tubules. In this group liver pathology is rarely a problem. Polycystic disease presenting in later childhood tends to have more severe liver involvement and less severe renal involvement. Patients frequently develop portal hypertension and gastrointestinal bleeding from varices. The renal cysts in these children may have a fusiform appearance similar to those of the infant or may have a more rounded contour. On T1-weighted spin-echo images, the high signal intensity within the cysts is due to the presence of subacute hemorrhage (methemoglobin).

Differential diagnosis includes the other causes of cystic renal disease: multicystic kidney, adult type polycystic disease, cystic renal tumors, and diseases such as tuberous sclerosis and Hippel-Lindau disease, in which renal cysts may be seen.

References

1. Dietrich RB, Kangarloo H. Kidneys in infants and children: evaluation with MR. *Radiology* 1986;159:215–221.
2. Demas B, Thurnher S, Hricak H. The kidney, adrenal gland and retroperitoneum. In: Higgins CB, Hricak H, eds. *Magnetic resonance of the body.* New York: Raven Press, 1987;373–401.
3. Hilpert PL, Friedman AC, Radecki PD, et al. MRI of hemorrhagic renal cysts in polycystic kidney disease. *AJR* 1986;146:1167–1172.

Submitted by: Rosalind B. Dietrich, M.B., Ch.B., Senior Editor.

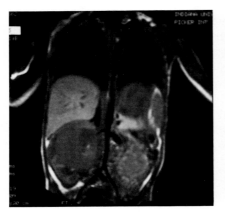

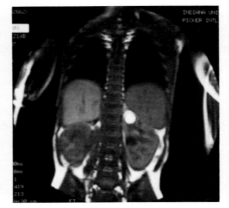

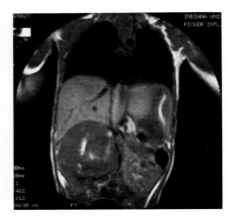

FIG. 89A. SE 500/16.   FIG. 89B. SE 500/16.   FIG. 89C. SE 500/16.

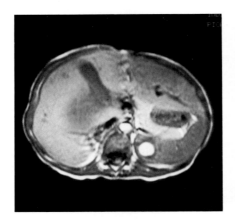

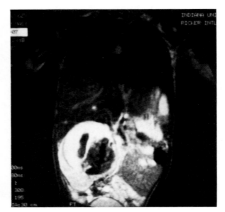

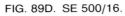

FIG. 89D. SE 500/16.   FIG. 89E. SE 2,000/80.

Clinical History

A 2-year-old white male with anorexia and abdominal pain and a right-sided abdominal mass.

Findings

Coronal (Figs. 89A–C) T1-weighted images show a very large mass lesion arising from the upper medial aspect of the right kidney. The mass is well defined (Figs. 89A and C) and clearly separate from the liver. Most of the mass is isointense with muscle, but a few areas of high signal intensity probably represent hemorrhage within the mass. The aorta (Fig. 89A) shows minimal displacement to the left and is patent.

The inferior vena cava (Fig. 89C) is displaced to the left by the mass. No tumor is seen within it. Note the normal inferior vena cava on the transverse image (Fig. 89D) and also note how difficult it is to clearly exclude hepatic invasion on the transverse image (Fig. 89D). T2-weighted image (Fig. 89E) shows marked increase in signal intensity from most of the lesion. Some areas are very low signal intensity and probably represent hemosiderin deposition in areas of old hemorrhage. Note an incidental well-defined cyst in the upper pole of the opposite kidney (Fig. 89B). The high signal on T1-weighted image indicates either hemorrhage or high protein content within this cyst.

Diagnosis

Classic Wilms' tumor of the right kidney without metastases to lymph nodes and without invasion of the inferior vena cava.

Discussion

Wilms' tumor is the most common tumor of the genitourinary tract in children and accounts for 10% of all malignancies in childhood. The tumors are usually large at presentation and often contain focal areas of hemorrhage and necrosis. Bilateral tumors occur in 10% of patients. Spread of tumor is into regional lymph nodes and liver and also by direct invasion of the renal vein into the inferior vena cava. Pulmonary metastases are common. Calcification of the tumors is unusual.

MR has the potential of replacing all other modalities for the evaluation of patients with suspected Wilms' tumor. It can evaluate the primary tumor mass and opposite kidney, inferior vena cava and liver, and regional lymph nodes. It may therefore replace CT, ultrasound, and liver/spleen scan in the evaluation of patients with Wilms' tumor. The classic MR findings are of a large mass involving the kidney. The mass is almost always well defined. Areas of necrosis and hemorrhage cause varied signal intensity on T1 and T2 pulse sequences.

Treatment is by surgical resection of the primary tumor followed by chemotherapy. Radiotherapy is utilized in patients in whom there is residual abdominal disease following surgery.

References

1. Cohen MD. Radiology of pediatric abdominal masses. Radiological Society of North America annual meeting, Pediatric Refresher Course Syllabus, Chicago, 1989;197–211.
2. Belt TG, et al. MRI of Wilms' tumor. Promise as the primary imaging method. *AJR* 1986;146:955–961.
3. Kangarloo H, et al. Magnetic resonance imaging of Wilms' tumor. *Urology* 1986;28:203–207.

Submitted by: Mervyn D. Cohen, M.B., Ch.B., Riley Hospital for Children, Indiana University Medical Center, Indianapolis, Indiana; Rosalind B. Dietrich, M.B., Ch.B., Senior Editor.

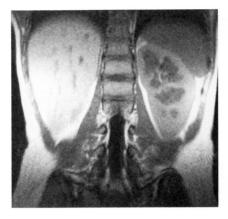

FIG. 90A. SE 286/16.

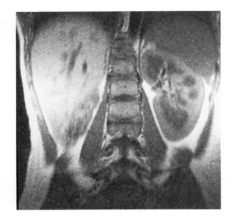

FIG. 90B. SE 286/16.

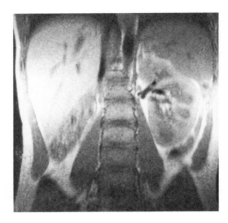

FIG. 90C. SE 286/16.

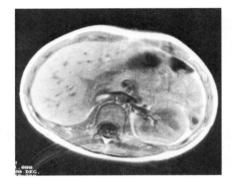

FIG. 90D. SE 389/16.

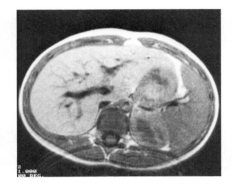

FIG. 90E. SE 389/16.

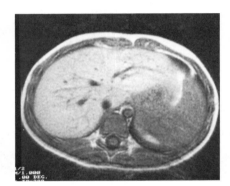

FIG. 90F. SE 389/16.

Clinical History

A 6-year-old boy with a history of one urinary tract infection.

Findings

T1-weighted coronal and axial images demonstrate the presence of the left kidney in the left renal fossa. It is enlarged in size (five vertebral bodies in length) but is otherwise unremarkable. The corticomedullary differentiation appears normal. The ipsilateral adrenal gland is also normal in size and configuration. On the right side, however, there is no evidence of a kidney in the renal fossa nor can an ectopic kidney be identified. The right adrenal gland is present but has an elongated configuration.

Diagnosis

Agenesis of the right kidney, discoid adrenal gland, and compensatory hypertrophy of the contralateral kidney.

Discussion

Unilateral agenesis of the kidney is occasionally seen and is thought to be due to a loss of the blood supply to the kidney *in utero*. Whenever a kidney is not identified within the renal fossa, it is important to thoroughly search for it in an ectopic location, either more inferiorly in the retroperitoneum or the pelvis. It is also important to fully evaluate the contralateral kidney to rule out the presence of fusion anomalies before confirming the diagnosis of renal agenesis.

When the kidney does not develop within the renal fossa, secondary effects are seen in the ipsilateral adrenal gland. It demonstrates an elongated discoid appearance instead of its usual triangular shape. The contralateral kidney frequently demonstrates compensatory hypertrophy.

Children with agenesis of the kidney may also have other anomalies of the urinary tract. In girls anomalies of the uterus and vagina may also be present.

When using MR to evaluate congenital anomalies of abdominal structures, multiplanar T1-weighted images are frequently all that is necessary. Additional T2-weighted images must be obtained, however, if congenital anomalies that are associated with an increased incidence of neoplasia are being evaluated.

References

1. Dietrich RB, Kangarloo H. Kidneys in infants and children: evaluation with MR. *Radiology* 1986;159:215–221.
2. Demas B, Thurner S, Hricak H. The kidney, adrenal gland and retroperitoneum. In: Higgins CB, Hricak H, eds. *Magnetic resonance imaging of the body.* New York: Raven Press, 1987;373–401.

Submitted by: Rosalind B. Dietrich, M.B., Ch.B., Senior Editor.

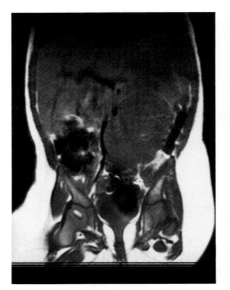

FIG. 91A. SE 700/20.

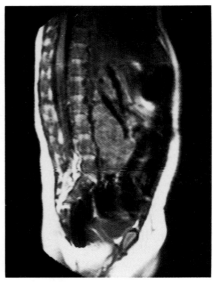

FIG. 91B. SE 800/26.

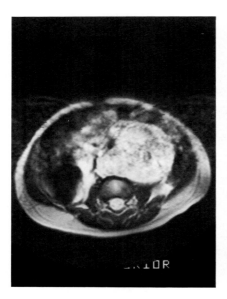

FIG. 91C. SE 2,000/80.

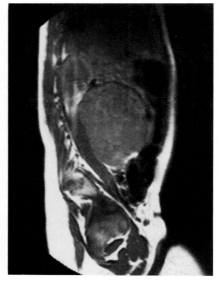

FIG. 91D. SE 800/26.

Clinical History

A 7-month-old male infant taken to his pediatrician for routine care. An abdominal mass was found on clinical examination.

Findings

There is a large, well-defined left-sided abdominal mass (Figs. 91A–D). The mass is of fairly homogeneous soft tissue intensity on the T1-weighted images and very high signal on the T2-weighted images. The mass is lying anterior to the left kidney, which appears normal. The aorta (Fig. 91A), superior mesenteric artery (Fig. 91B), and inferior vena cava (Fig. 91C) are all displaced by the mass, which is closely adherent to these vessels. The mass crosses the midline.

Diagnosis

Left sympathetic chain abdominal neuroblastoma.

Discussion

The abdominal mass is fairly nonspecific, and there are no definitive features to suggest the correct diagnosis. The mass is not arising from either adrenal gland. Both kidneys appear normal, excluding Wilms' tumor, hydronephrosis, multicystic dysplastic kidney, etc. The lesion is clearly solid and not cystic, excluding disorders such as duplication cyst, ovarian cyst, etc. Subtle calcification, identified on CT, was not imaged on MR. This CT finding does help in the differential diagnosis, suggesting neuroblastoma. The lack of any adjacent soft tissue abnormality is against an abscess as is the soft tissue intensity on the T1-weighted images. In a child of this age, an abdominal mass, with exclusion of the above-mentioned disorders, is most likely to be a neuroblastoma.

MR correctly identified the very close association of the tumor mass to several major abdominal blood vessels. It also correctly identified the lack of any invasion of these blood vessels. At surgery, because of the close association of the tumor with the major blood vessels, it was not possible to completely resect it.

References

1. Cohen MD. Radiology of pediatric abdominal masses. Radiological Society of North America annual meeting, Chicago, 1989;197–211.
2. Cohen MD, et al. The visualization of major blood vessels by magnetic resonance in children with malignant tumors. *Radiographics* 1985;5:441–455.
3. Cohen MD, et al. Magnetic resonance imaging of neuroblastoma. *AJR* 1984;143:1241–1248.

Submitted by: Mervyn D. Cohen, M.B., Ch.B., Riley Hospital for Children, Indiana University Medical Center, Indianapolis, Indiana; Rosalind B. Dietrich, M.B., Ch.B., Senior Editor.

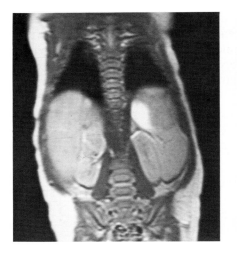

FIG. 92A. SE 2,500/30.

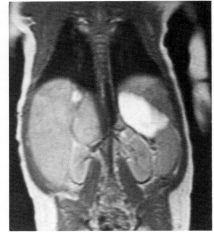

FIG. 92B. SE 2,500/30.

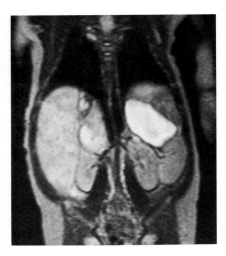

FIG. 92C. SE 2,500/80.

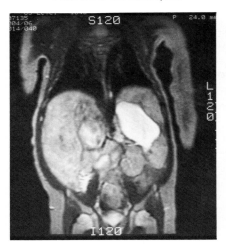

FIG. 92D. SE 2,500/80.

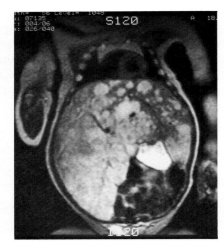

FIG. 92E. SE 2,500/80.

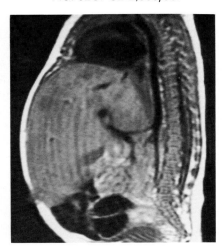

FIG. 92F. SE 500/20.

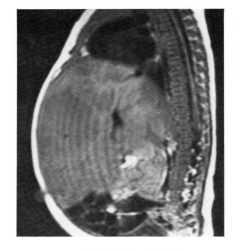

FIG. 92G. SE 500/20.

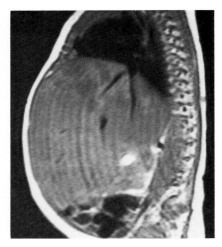

FIG. 92H. SE 500/20.

Clinical History

A 3-month-old girl with an enlarged liver.

Findings

Coronal proton density and sagittal T1-weighted images demonstrate a medium signal intensity, right adrenal mass displacing the right kidney inferiorly. The left kidney and adrenal gland appear normal. The aorta, IVC, and left renal vessels are displaced but not involved by the tumor, and there is no evidence of extension of the lesion into the spinal canal. The liver is enlarged and contains multiple discrete medium signal intensity lesions. The bone marrow of the vertebral bodies has diffuse low signal intensity. On coronal T2-weighted images, the liver lesions demonstrate high signal intensity as does the right adrenal lesion.

Diagnosis

Metastatic neuroblastoma (grade IV-S).

Discussion

Neuroblastoma is the most common abdominal neoplasm in childhood. It most frequently arises from the adrenal gland but may be seen anywhere along the sympathetic chain from the nasopharynx to the presacral region. Children with neuroblastoma may present with a palpable abdominal mass or symptoms referable to metastases as in those who complain of bone pain. Neuroblastoma is staged based on the local extent of the tumor and the presence or absence of metastases. Clinically, however, it is more important to determine if the lesion is operable or inoperable as surgery is the treatment of choice.

On MR images, neuroblastoma usually demonstrates medium signal intensity on T1-weighted images and high signal intensity on T2-weighted images. The role of MR in the evaluation of children with neuroblastoma includes identifying the organ of origin of the lesion, defining its extent and relationship to adjacent vessels, and evaluating for the presence of metastasis to the liver, bone marrow, or cortex. In this case the lesion is seen to originate from the right adrenal gland with evidence of metastasis to the liver and bone marrow (grade IV-S).

References

1. Dietrich RB, Kangarloo H, Lenarsky C, et al. Neuroblastoma: the role of MR imaging. *AJR* 1987;148:937–941.
2. Cohen MD, Weetman RM, Provisor AJ, et al. Magnetic resonance imaging of neuroblastoma with a 0.15T magnet. *AJR* 1984;143:1241–1244.

Submitted by: Rosalind B. Dietrich, M.B., Ch.B., Senior Editor.

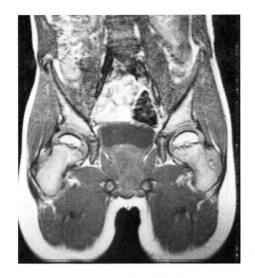

FIG. 93A. SE 900/20.

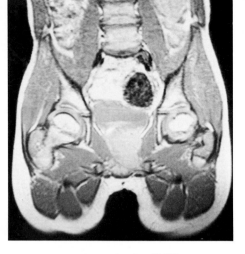

FIG. 93B. SE 2,100/20.

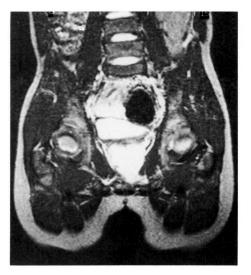

FIG. 93C. SE 2,100/80.

Clinical History

A 6-year-old white male with a history of difficulty in urination for several weeks.

Findings

There is a large soft tissue mass lesion in the region of the prostate gland. It is of similar intensity to muscle on the T1-weighted image (Fig. 93A) showing mild increase in signal intensity on spin density image (Fig. 93B) and marked increase in signal intensity on T2-weighted image (Fig. 93C). The lesion is moderately well defined on the T2-weighted image (Fig. 93C). There appears to be a patchy increase in signal intensity from the bladder wall, which is mildly thickened. The bones appear normal. No enlarged lymph nodes are identified.

Diagnosis

Prostatic rhabdomyosarcoma.

Discussion

Rhabdomyosarcoma comprises approximately 10% of childhood solid tumors. They can be found in almost any region of the body. In boys the prostate is a fairly common location. Metastasis is to lymph nodes, lung, liver, and bone. The tumors are usually well defined with signal intensity consistent with prolongation of T1 and T2 relaxation times as compared to normal soft tissue.

The location of the lesion in the region of the prostate gland is fairly characteristic for rhabdomyosarcoma as this is almost the only prostatic disorder found in children. Other pelvic tumors do, however, need to be considered in the differential diagnosis. Cystic lesions including teratoma can be excluded by the lack of fluid in this patient's lesion. The signal intensity on the T1-weighted image is greater than that of urine in the bladder above it. Pelvic neuroblastoma or Burkitt's lymphoma might appear very similar to this lesion as might a pelvic abscess.

References

1. Cohen MD, et al. Efficacy of magnetic resonance imaging in 139 children with tumors. *Arch Surg* 1986;121:522–528.
2. Bartolozzi C, et al. Rhabdomyosarcoma of the prostate: MR findings. *AJR* 1988;150:1333–1335.

Submitted by: Mervyn D. Cohen, M.B., Ch.B., Riley Hospital for Children, Indiana University Medical Center, Indianapolis, Indiana; Rosalind B. Dietrich, M.B., Ch.B., Senior Editor.

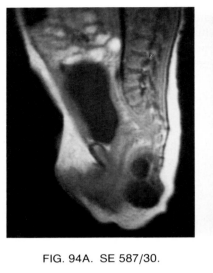

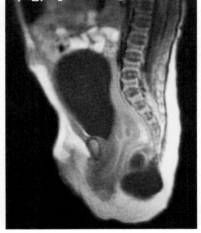

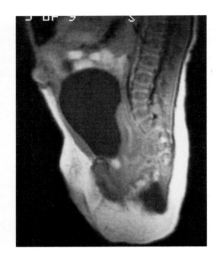

FIG. 94A. SE 587/30.

FIG. 94B. SE 587/30.

FIG. 94C. SE 587/30.

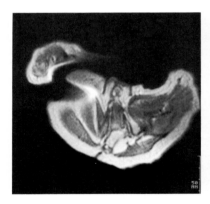

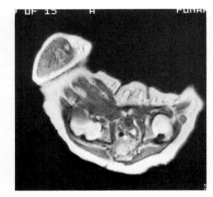

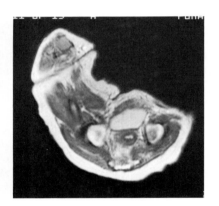

FIG. 94D. SE 2,000/85.

FIG. 94E. SE 2,000/85.

FIG. 94F. SE 2,000/85.

Clinical History

A 6-day-old girl presents with a mass palpable below the coccyx.

Findings

T1-weighted sagittal images demonstrate a mass situated between the rectum anteriorly and sacrum posteriorly and superiorly, but invading neither. The mass has low signal intensity and is septated. On T2-weighted images, it demonstrates inhomogeneous high signal intensity. The adjacent uterus appears prominent in size due to the effects of maternal estrogen stimulation that are normally still present in a female child of 6 days of age. The remainder of the pelvic structures and the spinal canal and cord appear normal.

Diagnosis

Sacrococcygeal teratoma.

Discussion

Sacrococcygeal teratoma is the most common presacral mass seen in children. It usually presents as a buttocks or perineal mass or secondary to pressure effects on adjacent structures. It is more frequently seen in girls and may be cystic, solid, or mixed in character. Differential diagnosis of a presacral mass in this age group includes anterior meningocele, rectal duplication, neuroblastoma, and lipoma.

The MR findings are characteristic of a septated, cystic, presacral mass. Of the above differential diagnoses, anterior meningocele, neuroblastoma, and lipoma can be excluded as the former would demonstrate an associated abnormality of the sacrum not seen in this case and the latter two would have different MR characteristics. A rectal duplication cannot be excluded on this examination.

References

1. Friedman AC, Pyatt RS, Hartman DS, Downey EF Jr, Olson WB. CT of benign cystic teratomas. *AJR* 1982;138:659–665.
2. Schey WL, Shkolnik A, White H. Clinical and radiologic considerations of sacrococcygeal teratomas: an analysis of 26 new cases and review of the literature. *Radiology* 1977;125:189–195.

Submitted by: Rosalind B. Dietrich, M.B., Ch.B., Senior Editor.

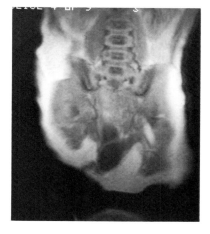

FIG. 94G. SE 649/30.

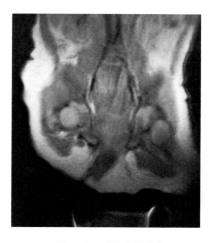

FIG. 94H. SE 649/30.

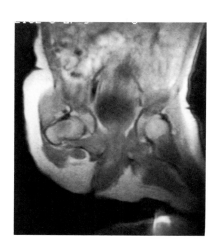

FIG. 94I. SE 649/30.

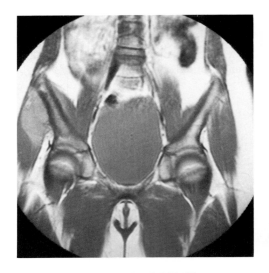

FIG. 95A. SE 2,033/20.

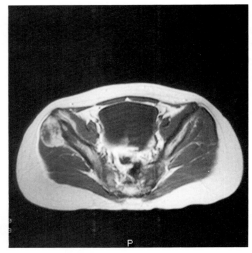

FIG. 95B. SE 1,300/20 with Gd-DTPA.

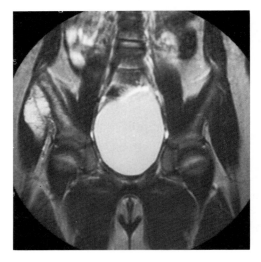

FIG. 95C. SE 2,033/80.

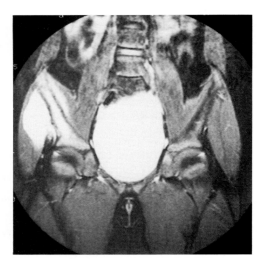

FIG. 95D. IR 2,133/150/30.

Clinical History

An 11-year-old girl who presented with pain in the right groin and hip following a fall from a horse. Clinical examination revealed fullness in the right gluteal area posterior to the right iliac crest.

Findings

Spin density image (Fig. 95A) shows soft tissue fullness lateral to the right iliac crest together with mild decrease in marrow signal intensity on this side as compared to the other side. There is also patchy increase in signal intensity from the cortical bone of the iliac wing on the right, as compared to the left. The cortex is also thickened. There is inhomogeneous enhancement of the mass lesion and bone marrow following gadolinium administration (Fig. 95B). T2-weighted image (Fig. 95C) and STIR images (Fig. 95D) taken before administration of gadolinium also show the soft tissue mass lesion with an increase in signal intensity in the bone marrow. Note that the soft tissue mass, particularly medial to the iliac wing, and the extensive involvement of the bone marrow are best appreciated on the STIR pulse sequence (Fig. 95D).

Diagnosis

Osteogenic sarcoma.

Discussion

Although osteogenic sarcoma is more common in the long bones, particularly around the knee joint, it can occur in the axial skeleton, and in this location the pelvic bones are a common site. Ewing's sarcoma is more common than osteogenic sarcoma in the pelvic bones, and there are no specific features in this patient to permit differentiation of these two tumors.

Infection should also be considered in the differential diagnosis. This will cause abnormal signal in the bone marrow, cortex, and soft tissue. The well-defined margins of the soft tissue abnormality are against infection.

In addition the patient had no clinical findings of infection.

It is extremely important in this patient to demonstrate abnormality in the entire iliac bone extending into the roof of the acetabulum. This was demonstrated far better on MR as compared to CT. In addition, on the MR, only the STIR sequence shows the full extent of the marrow abnormality. The importance of this finding is that the tumor cannot be resected without sacrificing the entire iliac bone and hip joint.

References

1. Cohen MD, et al. Magnetic resonance imaging of bone marrow disease in children. *Radiology* 1984;151:715–718.
2. Boyko OB, et al. Magnetic resonance imaging of osteogenic sarcoma and Ewing's sarcoma. *AJR* 1987;148:317–322.
3. Gillespy T, et al. Staging of intraosseous extent of osteosarcoma: correlation of preoperative CT and MR imaging with pathologic macroslides. *Radiology* 1988;167:765–767.
4. Jones BE, et al. MR appearances of childhood bone tumors. *AJR* 1989;153:202–203.

Submitted by: Mervyn D. Cohen, M.B., Ch.B., Riley Hospital for Children, Indiana University Medical Center, Indianapolis, Indiana; Rosalind B. Dietrich, M.B., Ch.B., Senior Editor.

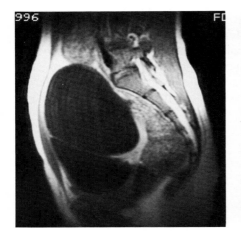

FIG. 96A. SE 300/18.

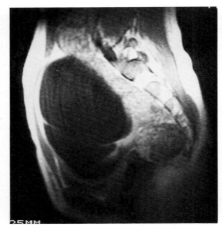

FIG. 96B. SE 300/18.

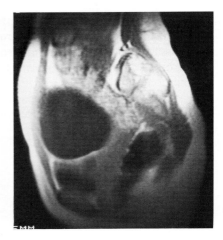

FIG. 96C. SE 300/18.

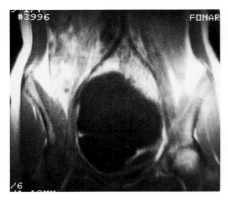

FIG. 96D. SE 300/18.

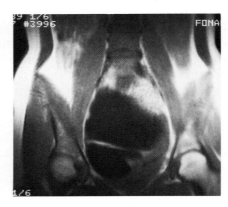

FIG. 96E. SE 300/18.

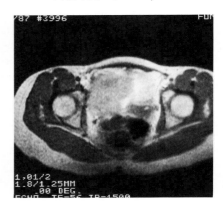

FIG. 96F. SE 1,500/56.

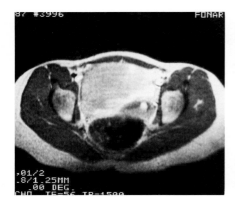

FIG. 96G. SE 1,500/56.

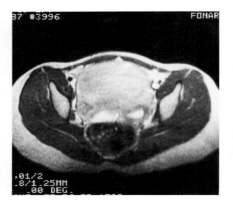

FIG. 96H. SE 1,500/56.

Clinical History

A 14-year-old girl with a history of increasing abdominal girth and constipation.

Findings

T1-weighted sagittal and coronal images demonstrate a large, well-defined, low signal intensity mass arising from the pelvis and extending superiorly into the abdomen. Septations are present within the mass. The mass is compressing but not involving the bladder anteriorly and the rectum posteriorly. There is no evidence of ascites.

On relatively T2-weighted axial images, the mass demonstrates high signal intensity. The uterus is displaced to the left by the mass but appears separate from it.

Diagnosis

Cystadenoma of the ovary.

Discussion

Ovarian tumors are uncommon in the pediatric age group, especially in children under 5 years of age. Older children most frequently present with pain, whereas younger children more frequently present following detection of an abdominal mass.

As in adults, the tumors may be of surface epithelium origin (adenomas and adenocarcinomas) or germ cell origin (teratomas, dysgerminomas, and gonadoblastomas) or be metastatic (lymphoma, leukemia, and neuroblastoma). In children, the most frequently seen lesions are teratomas, dysgerminomas, cystadenomas, and cystadenocarcinomas, embryonal carcinomas, and granulosa cell tumors.

As with other imaging modalities, MR is not always able to give a definitive diagnosis of the type of ovarian tumor present but can identify the lesions as being cystic, solid, or mixed in nature, thus narrowing the differential diagnosis. The differential diagnosis of cystic lesions involving the ovary includes ovarian cysts, abscesses, cystadenomas, and cystadenocarcinomas. When a septated, cystic lesion of this size is seen, cystadenoma or cystadenocarcinoma is the most likely diagnosis.

References

1. Reis RL, Koop CE. Ovarian tumors in infants and children. *J Pediatr* 1962;60:96–102.
2. Dooms GC, Hricak H, Tscholakoff D. Adnexal structures: MR imaging. *Radiology* 1986;158:639.
3. Hricak H. MRI of the female pelvis: a review. *AJR* 1986;146:1115–1122.
4. Dietrich RB, Kangarloo H. Pelvic abnormalities in children: assessment with MR imaging. *Radiology* 1987;163:367.

Submitted by: Rosalind B. Dietrich, M.B., Ch.B., Senior Editor.

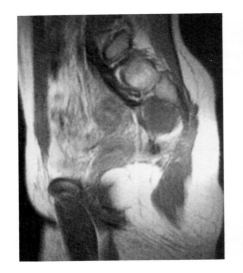

FIG. 97A. SE 500/30.

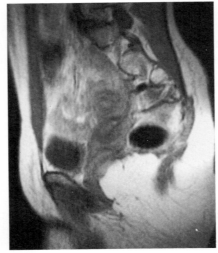

FIG. 97B. SE 500/30.

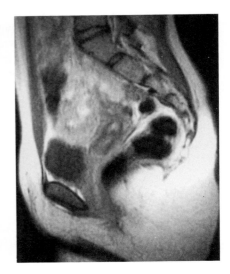

FIG. 97C. SE 500/30.

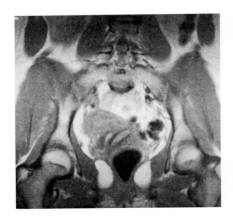

FIG. 97D. SE 600/30.

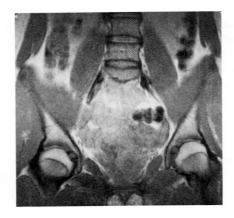

FIG. 97E. SE 600/30.

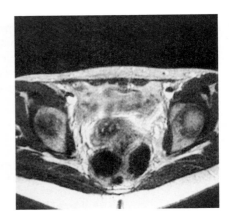

FIG. 97F. SE 2,000/85.

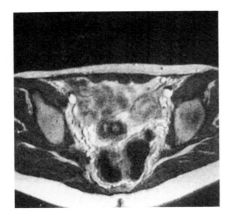

FIG. 97G. SE 2,000/85.

Clinical History

A 12-year-old girl with an abnormal pelvic ultrasound scan.

Findings

MR images demonstrate an abnormal configuration of the uterus. On coronal T1-weighted images, two uterine cavities are identified. On T2-weighted images, differentiation of the different layers of the uterus can be seen. There are two high signal intensity endometrial and endocervical signals seen and two low signal intensity junctional zones surrounding them. Between the junctional zones a medium signal intensity band of myometrial tissue is identified. The ovaries are in normal position and the other pelvic organs are unremarkable.

Diagnosis

Uterus didelphys.

Discussion

Abnormalities caused by incomplete fusion of the Müllerian ducts are numerous. When complete failure of fusion occurs, as in this case, two uteri, two cervices, and two vaginas are present (uterus didelphys). Incomplete fusion leads to the development of such lesions as bicornate uterus (single vagina and cervix with two uteri) and uterus septus (single vagina, cervix, and uterus with uterine septum). Occasionally in children with a double vagina, one half is imperforate.

These uterine abnormalities can frequently be diagnosed and differentiated using MR thus obviating the need for more invasive diagnostic procedures. In postpubertal girls, MR is able to differentiate didelphyc and bicornuate uteri from septate uteri. This is important clinically as the two anomalies require different surgical management. On axial T2-weighted images patients with bicornuate uteri will demonstrate a medium signal intensity strip of myometrium separating the two low signal intensity junctional zones that will not be seen in children with septate uteri.

Müllerian duct anomalies are also associated with a wide spectrum of genitourinary anomalies such as agenesis or malposition of the kidney.

References

1. Mintz MC, Thickman DI, Gussman D, Kressel HY. MR evaluation of uterine anomalies. *AJR* 1987;148:287–290.
2. Hricak H, Chun-Fang Chang Y. The female pelvis. In: Higgins CB, Hricak H, eds. *Magnetic resonance imaging of the body.* New York: Raven Press, 1987;403–431.

Submitted by: Rosalind B. Dietrich, M.B., Ch.B., Senior Editor.

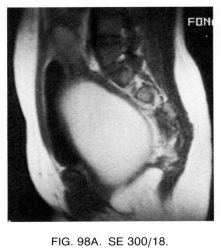

FIG. 98A. SE 300/18.

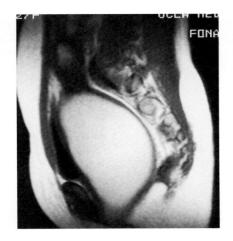

FIG. 98B. SE 300/18.

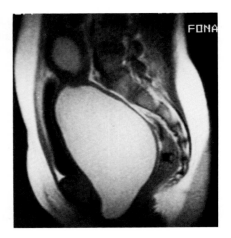

FIG. 98C. SE 300/18.

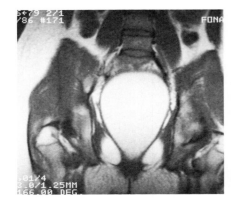

FIG. 98D. SE 300/28.

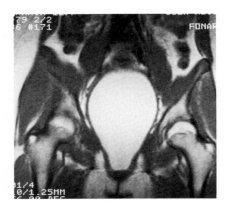

FIG. 98E. SE 300/28.

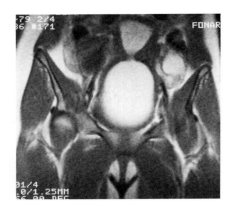

FIG. 98F. SE 300/28.

Clinical History

A 12-year-old girl presented with intermittent abdominal pain and amenorrhea.

Findings

T1-weighted sagittal and coronal images demonstrate a normal symphysis pubis. The bladder is compressed anteriorly but is otherwise unremarkable. Posteriorly the sacrum, coccyx, and rectum are unremarkable. The vagina and uterine cavity are distended and filled with high signal intensity fluid.

Diagnosis

Hematometrocolpos.

Discussion

Hematometrocolpos occurs when blood accumulates in the vagina and uterus because of the presence of congenital vaginal obstruction. The term hydrometrocolpos can only be used when secretions and no blood are present. Congenital vaginal obstruction may occur because of an imperforate hymen, vaginal diaphragm, atresia of the vagina or cervix, or because of a persistent urogenital sinus or cloaca. Patients with this abnormality most commonly present with an abdominal mass either in the newborn period when maternal hormonal influence is present or at puberty when the retained blood from menses accumulates cyclically and distends the vagina and uterus. At this age patients may also complain of vague abdominal pain or be investigated for primary amenorrhea. Associated anomalies include esophageal or duodenal atresia, malrotation, congenital heart disease, imperforate anus, or sacral agenesis.

The typical MR appearance is of a high signal intensity fluid collection, seen on both T1- and T2-weighted images, due to subacute hemorrhage distending the vagina and uterus. The dilated structures cause compression of the adjacent bladder and rectum. The sagittal plane best identifies the location of the fluid collection. In some instances the fluid collection may also extend into the adjoining fallopian tube, and then a tortuous and dilated fluid-filled fallopian tube can be seen extending into the abdomen. In children with Müllerian duct anomalies, hematometrocolpos may involve only a portion of the uterine cavity, and in these cases the adjacent nondistended portion of the uterus can be identified by MR.

Differential diagnosis is of other mass lesions arising in the pelvis. Those of ovarian origin would include ovarian teratomas, cystadenomas, or dysgerminomas. Lesions arising from structures of the pelvic sidewalls such as lymphoma, rhabdomyosarcoma, and neuroblastoma should also be considered. The majority of these lesions, however, would appear as solid lesions on MR images showing medium signal intensity on T1-weighted images and relatively high signal intensity on T2-weighted images. Cystic areas within the masses may be seen as areas of even higher signal on T2-weighted images in cystadenomas and teratomas. Areas of high signal intensity fat may be seen on T1-weighted images of teratomas, and of course any of the solid lesions containing areas of subacute hemorrhage would also demonstrate high signal intensity on T1-weighted images. None of these lesions, however, would demonstrate the characteristic MR appearance seen in hematometrocolpos.

References

1. Dietrich RB, Kangarloo H. Pelvic abnormalities in children: assessment with MR imaging. *Radiology* 1987;163:367–372.
2. Togashi K, Nishimura KZ, Itoh K, et al. Vaginal agenesis: classification by MR imaging. *Radiology* 1987;162:675–677.
3. Vinstein AL, Franken EA. Unilateral hematometrocolpos associated with agenesis of the kidney. *Radiology* 1972;102:625–628.

Submitted by: Rosalind B. Dietrich, M.B., Ch.B., Senior Editor.

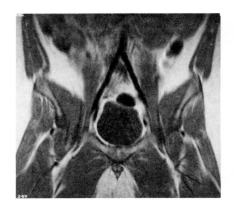

FIG. 99A. SE 693/30.

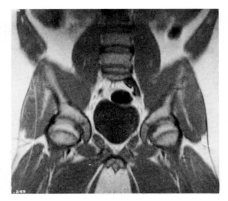

FIG. 99B. SE 693/30.

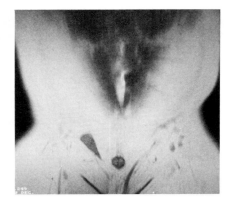

FIG. 99C. SE 693/30.

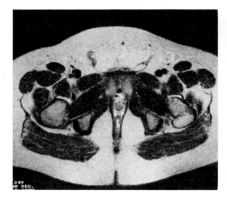

FIG. 99D. SE 2,000/85.

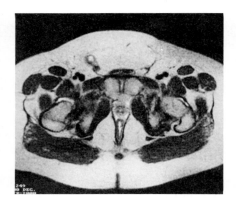

FIG. 99E. SE 2,000/85.

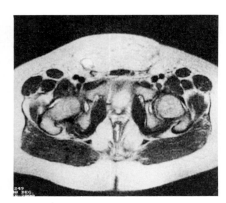

FIG. 99F. SE 2,000/85.

Clinical History

A 14-year-old boy with no palpable testis.

Findings

T1-weighted coronal images demonstrate an ovoid, medium signal intensity structure in the right inguinal canal that is outlined by the high signal intensity fat surrounding it. On T2-weighted axial images the same structure demonstrates high signal intensity and is surrounded by a lower signal intensity rim. No similar structure is identified on the contralateral side.

Diagnosis

Cryptorchidism (undescended inguinal testis).

Discussion

During intrauterine life, when the body cavity enlarges and parts of the mesonephros retract into the retroperitoneum, the testes, epididymis, and gubernaculum remain at the level of the internal inguinal ring. By birth most testes have completed their descent from this position into the scrotum.

Incomplete descent of the testis occurs in approximately 3% of births but only persists in 0.2%–0.7% of boys over 1 year of age. Evaluation of these children for localization of an undescended testis prior to surgery is frequently required if a testis cannot be palpated. Ultrasonography is usually the study performed initially. If ultrasonography is unsuccessful at locating the gonad, then MR should be performed.

The undescended gonad most commonly lies within the inguinal canal. If, however, it is positioned within the abdomen or pelvis it may be located adjacent to the lateral bladder wall, psoas muscle, or iliac vessels, in the retroperitoneum or superficial inguinal pouch. Rarely the gonad may be prepenile or perineal in position. Axial and/or coronal images obtained must of course cover this whole area.

Undescended and ectopically located testes have an increased susceptibility to torsion and trauma. As these patients may have impaired fertility and undescended testes may also undergo neoplastic change, it is important that they are located and surgically corrected.

Differential diagnosis of an ectopic testis in this location includes asymmetric muscle groups, lymphadenopathy, inguinal hernia, abscess, and tumors. When searching for ectopic gonads, T2-weighted sequences often add useful information, because on these sequences the appearance of the testis as a high signal intensity structure surrounded by a low signal intensity rim is very characteristic, helping to differentiate it from other masses.

References

1. Fritzsche PJ, Hricak H, Kogan BA, Winkler ML, Tanagho EA. Undescended testis: value of MR imaging. *Radiology* 1987;164:169–173.
2. Rajfer J, Walsh PC. Testicular descent. Normal and abnormal. Symposium on congenital anomalies of the lower genitourinary tract. *Urol Clin North Am* 1978;5:223.

Submitted by: Rosalind B. Dietrich, M.B., Ch.B., Senior Editor.

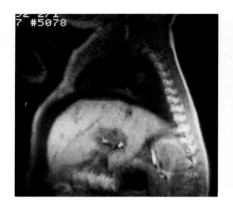

FIG. 100A. SE 300/18.

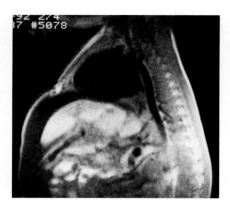

FIG. 100B. SE 300/18.

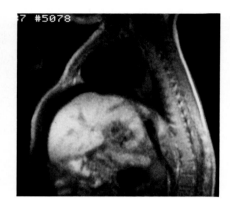

FIG. 100C. SE 300/18.

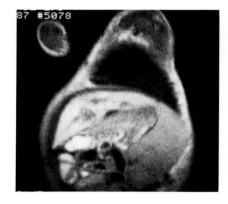

FIG. 100D. SE 300/18.

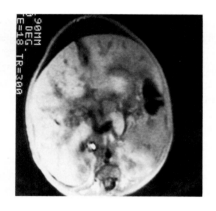

FIG. 100E. SE 300/18.

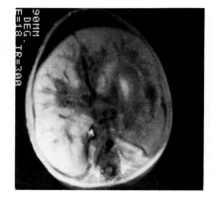

FIG. 100F. SE 300/18.

Clinical History

A 5-month-old boy who is a possible liver transplant candidate.

Findings

Sagittal and axial T1-weighted images through the liver reveal a small, shrunken liver demonstrating medium to high signal intensity. There is a large amount of low signal intensity ascites present surrounding the liver. The spleen appears enlarged and the kidneys are unremarkable. Within the liver, the portal vein is distended and has medium signal intensity on T1-weighted images and high signal intensity on T2-weighted images. There is a tubular structure situated between the medial and lateral segments of the left lobe of the liver that extends out of the liver anteriorly and passes toward the anterior abdominal wall. It demonstrates low signal intensity on both T1- and T2-weighted images, consistent with the appearance of a patent vessel.

Diagnosis

Chronic liver failure, splenomegaly, thrombosis of the portal vein, and recanalization of the umbilical vein.

Discussion

Causes of chronic liver failure in children include chronic active hepatitis, galactosemia, cystic fibrosis, Wilson's disease, and structural abnormalities of the biliary system such as biliary atresia and choledochal cysts. In the majority of instances, MR cannot identify the underlying cause of liver failure. Exceptions to this are when liver failure occurs secondary to abnormal deposition of substances within the liver that result in a change in its signal intensity. Decrease in signal intensity of the liver may be seen due to iron deposition in children with hemochromatosis or hemosiderosis secondary to multiple blood transfusions. Increase in signal intensity may be seen in diseases where there is lipid accumulation within the liver such as Wolman's disease.

In patients with chronic liver disease MR may be a useful adjunct to ultrasonography in identification of vessel patency or occlusion, especially in liver transplant candidates.

References

1. Stark DD, Goldberg HI, Moss AA, Bass NM. Chronic liver disease: evaluation by magnetic resonance. *Radiology* 1984;150:149.
2. Levy HM, Newhouse JH. MR imaging of the portal vein thrombosis. *AJR* 1988;151:283–286.

Submitted by: Rosalind B. Dietrich, M.B., Ch.B., Senior Editor.

CT scan of, 38, 64, 66
ventricles in, 36–38

U

Uterus
  didelphic, 224–225
  displacement of, 222–223
  hematometrocolpos, 226–227

V

Vascular malformations
  angiography of, 123
  cavernous hemangioma as, 122–123

classification of, 123
ICHs as, 82–84
innominate artery compression as,
  158–159

Vein of Galen
  CT scan of, 78, 81
  imaging of, 78–81

Ventricles
  ballooning of, 19
  dilation of, 18–19, 22–23
  enlargement of, 32, 45, 63
  ependymoma of, 114–115
  fourth, 104–105, 115
  in pachygyria, 22–23, 25

Ventricular septic defect (VSD),
  diagnosis of, 174–177
  pulmonary atresia and, 174–177
Vermis, absence of, 18–19
Vision loss
  in crainiopharyngioma, 58–59
  optic nerve glioma and, 60–61
  in subdural hematoma, 76–77
Von Recklinghausen's disease. *See*
  Neurofibromatosis

W

Wilms' tumor
  evaluation of, 209
  of kidney, 208–209